# EDUCATED AND TRAINED

*Recollections from the Diploma Nursing School Experience
1968 – 1971*

## Ila Minnick

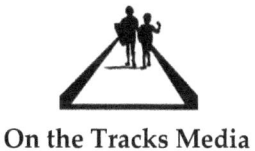

On the Tracks Media

Educated and Trained: Recollections from the Diploma Nursing School Experience, 1968-1971
Copyright © 2025 by Ila Minnick

All rights reserved. No part of this book may be reproduced or transmitted in any form or by any means, electronic or mechanical, including photocopying, recording, or any information storage and retrieval system, except in the case of brief passages embodied in critical reviews or articles, without permission from the author: Tminn10004@aol.com

Printed in the United States of America.
ISBN: 979-8-9869449-6-8

Interior Design: Rick Lindholtz for On the Tracks Media

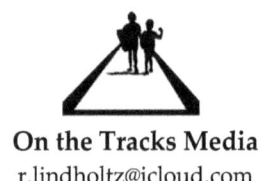

On the Tracks Media
r.lindholtz@icloud.com

10   9   8   7   6   5   4   3   2   1

# Acknowledgments

I gratefully acknowledge the following individuals for their contributions to this book:

Debra Arvidson, one of my dearest friends, thank you for meeting the challenge of accurately recalling the events, culture, and practice from your diploma school of nursing experience.

My cousins Doretta Hilst Irwin and Mary Judith Irwin Estes, for spending the day with me researching Mennonite's history. Thank you for making a tedious task lighter and for the opportunity to spend time with you and enjoy your company.

Linda Coyle, for generously sharing her expertise during the editing process. Her thoughtful insights enhanced the clarity and quality of this book.

Dale Curtin, a friend and skilled photographer, for creating the cover photo. His talent and eye for detail captured my vision for the cover photo and brought it to life.

I am grateful to the Mennonite College of Nursing at Illinois State University staff for warmly welcoming me to the college, providing a guided tour of the simulation area, and granting access to their historical archives.

And finally, I thank God for leading me to Mennonite.

# Dedication

It is with heartfelt gratitude that I dedicate this book to my family.

To Terry, my wonderful husband of 54 years, I want to express my gratitude for your unwavering support and encouragement. I love you, and I am grateful you have been by my side all these years.

To my children, Heather and Ryan, who survived "heart call", trauma call, first call, second call, administrative call, the night shift, and long hours. You endured hamburger helper, carry-out pizza, skillet lasagna, and most likely a weekly run to McDonald's. You have stood by me and loved me unconditionally. I love you and thank God for you every day.

To my son-in-law, Aaron, and daughter-in-law, Tiffany, you are God's precious gift to our family, and we thank Him for bringing you into our lives.

To my beautiful grandchildren, thank you for bringing me abundant joy. It's such a blessing to have you with us. God has a plan for your life.

# Table of Contents

HISTORICAL PERSPECTIVE: A BRIEF HISTORY OF NURSING .. 1

MY NURSING JOURNEY BEGINS ........................................................ 15

NURSING EDUCATION BEGINS ........................................................ 20

FRESHMAN YEAR 1968-1969 ................................................................ 45

JUNIOR YEAR 1969 – 1970 ...................................................................... 98

SENIOR YEAR 1970-1971 ..................................................................... 119

GRADUATION AND MOVING ON .................................................... 141

EPILOGUE .............................................................................................. 146

REFERENCES ........................................................................................ 148

# About the Author

Ila Minnick's half-century nursing career began with a rigorous and memorable diploma program in the late 1960s. In her memoir, Educated and Trained, she invites readers into a world of white caps, pristine uniforms, and bustling hospital corridors – a world where students were molded into nurses through discipline, compassion, and commitment

Drawing on her research, personal experiences, and memories, Ila reflects on what it meant to train in an era of hospital–based nursing education, when students lived in nurses' dorms and learned by doing. Her stories celebrate the friendships, challenges, and growth that defined her student years and laid the foundation for a lifelong profession in patient care.

After graduation, Ila went on to specialize in operating room nursing, where she served in many hospitals, large and small, mentored novice nurses, and witnessed the evolution of healthcare firsthand. Today, she shares her experiences to honor the legacy of diploma nurses and preserve a vital chapter in nursing history.

# Introduction

Some years ago, while on an outing with my daughter, she asked a thought-provoking question. If I had it to do over again, would I choose a career in nursing? Today, my answer would be a resounding "yes". But at that time, working in a stressful administrative role, navigating political minefields, and facing complex challenges while putting in long hours, I had to think about it. How would my career path have looked if I weren't a nurse? I began to review several options with her, all resulting in a negative response. Sales? No. Teaching? No. Marketing? No. Business? No. Anything involving math? Definitely not. At the end of this review, I concluded that yes, I would indeed choose nursing all over again.

So, why exactly did I pursue a career in nursing? It is certainly not the salary or the prestige. It is not a glamorous profession, often thankless, occasionally hostile, and intermittently frustrating, fraying the most solid of nerves. The work is physically and emotionally hard, sometimes grueling, at times unrelenting, and carries the potential for long hours. Yet it drew me like a magnet. And having done so, I have been privileged to experience the satisfaction and rewards of service to others.

I am not sure I chose nursing but rather, nursing chose me. I believe God called me to provide healing and comfort to His children. I have been uniquely privileged to witness the beginning and the end of life. I have been present when a baby took his or her first breath and marveled at the miracle of birth. Standing beside the patient as they breathed their last, I have learned that the line between life and death is often an imperceptible veil. And because of this, I pause to contemplate eternity and the Lord's gift of eternal life.

Following a brief history of nursing, the pages that follow chronicle my journey through my diploma nursing education, enriched by memorable personal stories. This education launched a 51-year nursing career spanning eight states, twelve organizations, and roles from staff nurse to Educator, Nurse Manager, Director, and Vice President of Nursing. As I walked up the Mennonite Hospital School of Nursing steps on that August day in 1968, I could never have imagined my professional journey for the next half a century. The Lord wove a golden thread of His presence throughout my career and life, and He never let go. And for that, I am most grateful.

# 1

# Historical Perspective: A Brief History of Nursing

As someone who enjoys history, I was interested in the historical origin of my profession. Curiosity drove me to the foundation and roots of my career. When, where, and how did the nursing profession begin? Medical care administered by physicians can be traced to ancient times, but the nurse's role is not as clear.

Although the ill and infirm have received care since ancient times, the nursing profession was not formally established until the nineteenth century. History shows that the earliest "healers" were witch doctors who relied on available remedies such as plants and minerals. Christianity influenced the development of nursing due to the Christian belief in self-sacrifice and serving others as a demonstration of love and obedience to God. Given this Christian influence, we should not be surprised that it was nuns who provided early documented care to the sick. The nuns profoundly influenced the profession including the nursing uniform itself.

Historical accounts center mainly around European and Asian countries. The growth of European-sponsored 17th-century expeditions worked to establish nursing in the New World. When America was founded, there were no trained nurses or physicians to care for the British colonists. As exploration grew, the early settlers to the United States included individuals known to be skilled in caring for the sick.

During this time, nursing care for the sick was provided by female family members who attended births and cared for the ill and dying in the home. For those individuals without a family to care for them, almshouses or poorhouses were established to house, feed, and care for the poor. Although the initial intent was to provide a charitable place to care for the poor, destitute, and sick, in reality, the almshouses were filthy, poorly maintained, and poorly funded with inadequate food and sanitation. The untrained inmates who provided the care were often lazy and unsavory. The original intent of almshouses was blurred as they became a catch-all for community outcasts. The earliest hospitals were established in these almshouses. As the city's first permanent almshouse, Bellevue Hospital, New York City, became the first public hospital in the United States in 1811 (Hehman, Keeling, & Kirchgessner, 2018).

Government leaders in Philadelphia were among the first to recognize the impossibility of delivering appropriate care in almshouses. Through the efforts of Benjamin Franklin and Dr. Thomas Bond, the Pennsylvania Hospital opened in 1752 to care for the sick (Hehman, Keeling, & Kirchgessner, 2018). The hospital was staffed by only three nurses. For over 100 years, untrained women and men provided the nursing care until a training school for nurses was established in 1883. Before that time, three training schools for nurses were opened in 1873. Early nineteenth-century "respectable" women did not pursue nursing because nurses were typically from lower social classes, considered outcasts with very bad reputations (Hallett, 2010). That began to change toward the mid-nineteenth century when working-class women pursued nursing to make a living. Women of higher society took a more philanthropic approach, viewing nursing as a charitable way to serve others (Hallett, 2010).

    Florence Nightingale helped transform the profession of nursing from that of downtrodden outcasts to respectable contributors to healthcare. Although she came from a wealthy family, she felt a divine calling to become a nurse. Because nursing was considered a profession for women of poor reputation and social status, her parents opposed her decision. However, she was undeterred by their opposition. Considered the founder of modern nursing, Florence Nightingale, born in 1820, was also an excellent statistician, English social reformer, and writer (Wikipedia, 2024). She is one of the most famous women of modern times (Hallett, 2010). Her skill as a statistician served her well. She used her statistical acumen to impact care in military hospitals by improving sanitation. She applied her statistical knowledge by keeping detailed, accurate records that validated the effectiveness of her care. She then correlated her patient care interventions to the improved mortality rates. During the Crimean War, which began in 1854, Nightingale was asked by the British Secretary of War to provide nursing services for the soldiers in the Turkish military hospital. Her expertise was sought to address the high mortality rate the hospital was experiencing. After receiving the request, she assembled a team of 38 nurses who traveled with her to Scutari, Turkey, where she trained these nurses to care for the hospitalized soldiers. Upon finding the hospital's dreadful, unsanitary conditions, she used her influence to draw attention to the plight of the soldiers. As a result, she was allowed to reorganize the hospital by training nurses to provide a higher level of skill to the soldiers. A focus on hygiene and improved living standards resulted in a dramatic decrease in the soldiers' death rate. Because Florence made rounds on the soldiers at night using light from her lantern to navigate the hospital wards, she became known as "the Lady with the Lamp" (Wikipedia, 2024).

A strong advocate for formal structured training for nurses, Florence Nightingale argued for an educated nursing workforce with patient care driven by standards of practice. The customary practice had nurses serving as apprentices in hospitals without formal education (Selanders and Crane, 2010). In 1860, she established the Nightingale Training School in London, the first secular nursing school in the world (Wikipedia, 2024).

Nightingale's books, *Notes on Hospital* and *Notes on Nursing* stressed the importance of morality and discipline while contributing to the practical training of nurses (Nurse Groups, 2018). Because of her upper-society Victorian background and her commitment to caring for the sick, Nightingale successfully transformed the prior unsavory career into an honorable profession for women. She also advocated for women's freedom to pursue the career of their choice.

The Civil War confirmed the demand for additional nurses to care for the sick and injured while underscoring the need for physical areas to house these patients. Although the nurses were expected to care for the injured war casualties, neither the Union nor the Confederacy nurses were trained to do so. The need for educated and trained nurses was becoming acutely obvious.

To address this void, Abraham Lincoln created the U.S. Sanitary Commission and appointed Nurse Dorothea Dix as superintendent of women nurses in the army to manage all Union female nurses. Because Dix had no official corps of nurses, 100 women were enlisted to receive a month's training from physicians at Bellevue and New York Hospitals (Hehman, Keeling, & Kirchgessner, 2018, p. 31). Due to the Civil War's magnitude, scores of additional nurses were required to meet the need to care for the wounded soldiers. Undeterred, these women faced disdain from their physician counterparts while they dealt with a lack of adequate nutrition for their patients, dismal sanitary conditions, lack of supplies, incompetent help, and long working hours, not to mention the emotional toll. These new nursing recruits worked tirelessly to gain the respect of the physicians, to organize and clean the wards, and to secure proper food and supplies. Nurse Clara Barton transported supplies to the battlefield, provided care to the men in the field, and was credited with starting the American Red Cross. By the end of the Civil War, 3,000 northern and 1,000 southern women had served as nurses. They were credited with organizing and improving the hospitals in both the North and the South. As a result, their success was counted as evidence that validated the benefits provided by trained nurses (Hehman, Keeling, & Kirchgessner, 2018).

The 1893 World's Fair in Chicago introduced Americans to hamburgers, the Ferris wheel, the Pledge of Allegiance, and the idea of higher education for nurses (Selanders, 2010). Selanders noted that nurse leaders of the time — including Nightingale, who did not attend the conference but had her last significant paper presented there — argued for an educated workforce with standards of practice, as opposed to one in which nurses served as apprentices in hospitals, which was customary at the time (Selanders, 2010).

World War II dramatically influenced nursing with significant changes in science, medicine, and the hospital industry. Attitudes shifted regarding working women when the soldiers returned from the war. Women who had been in the workforce transitioned to being housewives as the men returned to their jobs. The post-war culture reflected women's desire to remain home and care for the family. Because nursing was a predominantly female profession, nurses also returned to their homes and did not pursue careers in nursing at previous numbers, leading to a declining number of nurses (Hehman, Keeling, & Kirchgessner, 2018).

During the 1940s and 1950s, medical science and technology rapidly advanced, necessitating even more nurses. Specialties within medicine and the healthcare system meant that nurses were needed to support larger numbers of acutely ill patients. Medicine was advancing in cardiovascular medicine, cancer, kidney disease, as well as dialysis, mental health, and other specialties. Advances in cardiovascular and thoracic surgical techniques produced higher acuity procedures leading to acutely ill patients requiring higher levels of nursing care. These procedures heightened the need for additional acute care beds requiring larger post-anesthesia care units and intensive care beds. Skilled surgical and perioperative nurses were needed for a growing surgical volume, increasingly complex procedures, and higher acuity patients. Medical advances translated into the need for additional hospitals and the expansion of existing hospitals. The Hill-Burton Act of 1946 dramatically increased the number of hospital beds and highlighted the existing nursing shortage.

As the geographical model of the hospital ward evolved, private and semi-private patient rooms replaced larger multi-patient wards. This shift necessitated a change in the staffing model and heightened the need for even more nurses. The nursing supply was not meeting nursing demand.

The nurse's role was also expanding as increased nursing autonomy took hold. The advent of antibiotics and new medications changed medical care. Nurses were now required to prepare and administer a broader scope of medications and to monitor the patient's response to those medications (Hehman, Keeling, & Kirchgessner, 2018).

Adding to these challenges, nurses typically worked longer work weeks than other professions. While forty-hour work weeks were considered normal for most professions, nurses were expected to work well over 40 hours per week. In addition to the long hours, nursing salaries did not match the work or the demands placed on nurses. As a result, women either left the nursing workforce or avoided entering it (Hehman, Keeling, & Kirchgessner, 2018).

Attempts by the healthcare industry to adjust included "changes in nursing service administration, increased use of licensed practical nurses, and the establishment of associate degree programs in nursing" (Hehman, Keeling, & Kirchgessner, 2018, p. 296). All of this led to dramatic changes in the practice and education of nurses. Education was beginning to shift from a training model to a collegiate model, which meant that students would no longer serve as "staff" for hospitals. The new model emphasized that nursing students were just that, students. Hospitals could no longer depend on the students to staff their wards. The transition to four-year college/university baccalaureate education and two-year associate degree programs began the move away from the three-year hospital-based diploma programs that I experienced. As diploma programs closed, nursing students were unavailable to "staff" the hospital. The primary role of the nursing student became to learn rather than serve as hospital staff.

One of my best friends, Debbie Arvidson, shared her student experience staffing a hospital unit at a diploma school of nursing. She said during her second-year rotation, she was placed in charge of an entire Oncology unit housing approximately 20 patients. She was instructed to "call the nursing supervisor" if she needed help. She recalls that although her instructors were present in the hospital, they did not provide adequate supervision to the individual students. Adding to the challenge, the staff nurses hid when one of the more intense and vocal neurosurgeons rounded on his patients, leaving Debbie to round with the surgeon alone. Spoiler alert – this surgeon was to become one of our favorites when we later worked with him in the operating room at another facility. Although he could be intimidating, he was a brilliant and accomplished surgeon who was actually quite kind and humorous. Ultimately, Debbie and I forged a meaningful relationship of camaraderie and mutual respect with him. I guess he is responsible for the title of this book because he was the physician who asked me if I was educated or trained.

As a student in charge of that unit, she experienced her first patient death when one of her patients died of cancer. She recalls the husband standing outside the patient's room crying because his wife had died. He shared that he also had cancer and realized that he would die in the same way his wife had died. The lack of instructor supervision made Debbie feel ill-equipped and helpless to handle this situation. As a 20-year-old woman and young nursing student, she lacked the necessary skills to help this man as he experienced acute grief. She recalls subsequent experiences where she assumed responsibilities beyond her educational preparation.

The demand for nurses continued to grow while the supply pool could not meet that demand. Ancillary staff such as nursing assistants, orderlies, and Licensed Practical Nurses (LPN) grew. The team nursing care delivery model was born when nursing administrators were forced to develop a different model to deliver care. Patient care was administered as a team, with the ancillary staff focused on the bedside care of bathing, ambulating, toileting, feeding, and taking patient vitals. In addition to routine bedside care, LPNs could change dressings and provide wound care. The Registered Nurse (RN) was responsible for the more complex care that only an RN could provide. The nurse's scope of practice included coordinating patient care by leading the patient care team, administering medication, rounding with the physicians, monitoring the patient's response to medication, illness, and treatment, and communicating pertinent information to the physician.

In the team nursing model, registered nurses served as team leaders and coordinated patient care. A team consisting of the RN as team leader, LPNs, nursing assistants, and orderlies was assigned a certain number of patients on the ward. The team provided complete care within their scope of practice for those patients. The ancillary staff was responsible for bedside care while the RN coordinated that care, administered medications, and completed treatments as ordered. Each unit had a Head Nurse (called Nurse Managers today) in charge of the entire unit. A charge nurse for each shift rounded with the physicians, reviewed the physicians' orders, and communicated pertinent information to the team. Some nurses struggled with this change as responsibility shifted from bedside care to administrative tasks (Hehman, Keeling, & Kirchgessner, 2018). The 1950s saw the advent of progressive patient care areas and "step-down units". This model focused on the individual patient's needs as we began seeing patients progress from critical care areas to step-down units for discharge home (Hehman, Keeling, & Kirchgessner, 2018).

**1960's**

The 1960s were a time of political turmoil for the nation. The Vietnam War ramped up, resulting in unrest throughout the country, especially on college campuses. Increasing tension caused turmoil, dissension, and unrest. Although somewhat removed, Mennonite nursing students were certainly aware of the protests occurring on the Illinois State University campus. Emotions were raw, and tempers easily flared. When protestors attempted to remove the American flag from several areas of the Illinois State University college campus, my future husband and his roommates submitted an editorial in support of the American flag to the college newspaper. Publication of that editorial resulted in Terry and his friends receiving threatening phone calls from numerous anonymous sources. It was an unsettling experience.

At the same time, the nursing profession was experiencing its own challenges. With changes in technology and care delivery, nurses' roles were evolving, making it sometimes difficult to articulate the exact role of the RN. In a 1961 *American Journal of Nursing* article, Barbara Schutt described the biggest problem in nursing. She stated, "The profession was grappling with its boundaries, its role in the healthcare system, its overall identity – one that would separate it from medicine and social work" (Hehman, Keeling, & Kirchgessner, 2018, p. 309). Changes to the nursing profession would be driven by the "rise of Coronary Care units, new technology, increasing medical specialization, and the inception of the nursing roles of clinical nurse specialist and nurse practitioner" (Hehman, Keeling, & Kirchgessner, 2018, p. 310). All of these factors broadened nurses' scope of practice and autonomy, moving skills formerly performed by physicians to nurses. By providing care for the elderly and poor, Medicare and Medicaid legislation also impacted the healthcare system and, ultimately, nurses.

To address the need for care in underserved populations, Nurse Practitioner (NP) programs continued to grow into the 1970s. Increased specialization occurred in these roles with the growth of Pediatric Nurse Practitioner education. Nurses' scope of practice continued with increasing autonomy and transition of additional complex skills from physicians to nurses.

## 1970's

From 1965 to 1973, nurses served in the Vietnam War. Because women were not drafted, female nurses enlisted to serve and experienced the trauma and challenging living conditions associated with war. A monument near the Vietnam Memorial in Washington, DC, honors the nurses who served in that war.

As recognition of the value of Nurse Practitioners grew, so did the education and specialization of these roles. The Neonatal Nurse Practitioner role was the latest specialty in the 1970s. This expanded role allowed Nurse Practitioners to assume skills and responsibilities formerly completed by residents and physicians.

**1980s to 2000**

The emergence of AIDS in 1981 had a profound impact on healthcare in our nation and also in the world. Economic indicators challenged healthcare. With the 1980s recession came economic changes that reduced the cost of healthcare. "Unrestrained hospital spending, advances in technology, and an aging population" (Hehman, Keeling, & Kirchgessner, 2018, p. 332) drove rising healthcare costs, which outpaced economic growth during this era.

Changes in government hospital reimbursement exacerbated the nursing shortage as the Diagnosis-Related Group (DRG) classification was introduced in 1983 (Hehman, Keeling, & Kirchgessner, 2018). Hospitals were forced to trim their budgets, and as personnel are the biggest drivers of the budget, nursing positions were cut. At the same time, patient care was transitioning to the outpatient setting, resulting in patients with higher acuity occupying inpatient beds. Critical care beds increased to accommodate sicker patients. Nurses were challenged to deliver a high standard of care with fewer resources. Nurse salaries were not competitive with other occupations, which fueled the nursing shortage.

Nurses' outward appearance was beginning to change. The nursing uniform transitioned from all white to scrubs for cleanliness and to attract more men into the profession. Although I can't substantiate this in literature, I was told that because the nursing cap was considered a symbol of subservience to physicians, nurses would no longer wear it.

## 21st Century

The 21st Century saw nurses responding to a terrorist attack on September 11, 2001, as well as serving in the Iraq War, facing challenges during Hurricane Katrina, caring for patients during the severe Haiti earthquake in 2010, and responding to the more recent COVID pandemic.

A quarter of the way through the 21st Century, nursing's importance and significance in the healthcare arena continue to grow and expand. Nurses are integral to healthcare in all aspects of society – acute care hospitals, outpatient settings, the community, offices, clinics, and anywhere healthcare is delivered. Nurses gained increasing autonomy and knowledge, taking a prominent position on the healthcare stage. They work side by side with physicians, staff nurse-run clinics, work independently as midwives, serve as first assistants in the operating room, and provide care for the underserved. As the demand for nurses has grown, salaries have begun reflecting this need. Advanced practice nurses have demonstrated their value and work alongside physicians and other healthcare providers to care for the population.

The 21st century is seeing a growing number of males entering nursing. According to a March 2023 article by Nurse Journal, the number of male nurses has increased by 10 to 15% during the past 40 years and shows no indication of slowing down (Nurse Journal, 2023). They suggest that opportunity and job security are the major drivers of this increase in male nurses.

Our role as nurses continues to grow and evolve. We enjoy a greater scope of practice with increasing autonomy. I suspect our nursing ancestors could not have imagined the current role of today's nurse. Although the future of nursing looks promising, the ultimate purpose of this book is not to contemplate a future status. For now, please join me on my journey as I recall and reminisce about my nursing education and training over half a century ago.

# 2

## My Nursing Journey Begins

*Jeremiah 29:11 For I know the plans I have for you, declares the Lord, plans to prosper you and not to harm you, plans to give you a hope and a future.*

I am unable to recall a time when I did not want to be a nurse. I am uncertain what influences a child to decide on a specific career at a young age, but that was certainly me. An unseen force propelled me into medical things. I was the child with the toy doctor set and the toy nurse set, fixing my dolls, bandaging their limbs, taking their blood pressure, and giving them shots. And in 1960, I loved watching Ben Casey every Monday night. Never mind that Vince Edwards, who played Dr. Casey, was extremely handsome; I only hoped to catch a glimpse of the operating room during one of the surgery scenes.

I would like to say that I had a servant's heart, creating a desire to care for people who were ill and suffering. I would like to say that I unselfishly wished to ease that suffering. However, that was not the case for me. Quite simply, I found the medical world fascinating, and my curiosity drove me to it. I found the human body fascinating – how the anatomical components fit perfectly together with its intricate and complex physiology. In Psalms 139:14, the psalmist describes us as fearfully and wonderfully made, stating that the Lord's works are wonderful. In verse 15, he says that our frame was not hidden from God when we were made in the secret place, and we were woven together in the depths of the earth. We are a miracle from the Lord, and I was drawn to learn and experience more of God's miraculous creation. Although my initial motives were less than altruistic, as my education and career progressed and I had a chance to enter the world of the sick and suffering, I developed a heartfelt desire to serve and care for people.

I was especially fascinated by the surgical world, the mysterious operating room that one could only enter with specific qualifications and preparation. The first stirring occurred in 1955 at the age of four or five. My parents took me to Pekin Memorial Hospital's open house for their newly constructed six-story addition. My only recollection is standing outside the door of the huge operating room. I was mesmerized by the large light, the stainless-steel tables and bed, and the anesthesia machine, marveling at the sheer size and complexity of the room. This world held a fascination for me. In 1955, at the age of five, I was to experience this world first-hand when my tonsils were removed at that hospital in that department. I remember everyone dressed in white, the doctor greeting me, and the pungent smell of ether as I drifted off.

In 1959, at the age of nine, because the first tonsillectomy was botched, I underwent a second one at Methodist Hospital in Peoria, Illinois, with Dr. Sargent Howard. A defining moment occurred shortly after I arrived in the surgery department. While lying on the gurney outside the operating room awaiting my turn, a very kind nurse approached, took my hands, and spoke to me. She introduced herself as Thelma and said she would be with me during my operation. She told me how to breathe in the ether, and her kindness helped ease my fear. As I was being anesthetized, she stood beside me holding my hands. From that moment on, I wanted to be Thelma, a nurse in the operating room, participating in that world. The Lord was weaving a golden thread that would carry me through my life. Although that surgery was a traumatic ordeal, I knew I wanted to be like Thelma. At age nine, I knew I wanted to work in the operating room. That desire seldom wavered; my course was established. My fascination with the world of surgery continues to this day, over 50 years after receiving my nursing diploma.

In 1964, at 14 years of age, I was eligible to participate in the Candy Striper volunteer program at Pekin Memorial Hospital in Pekin, Illinois. Known for their red and white striped pinafore outfits resembling candy canes, Candy Stripers have volunteered in hospitals for 70 years. Being a Candy Striper allowed me to work alongside nurses and other healthcare professionals. Working amidst the sights, sounds, and smells of the healthcare world reinforced my desire to become part of it. During the summer months, I volunteered one or two mornings a week, and during school, I worked once a month on Saturdays. I recall feeling excited and proud to work inside the hospital. After working 100 hours, I received my cap. I was very proud of that cap because it felt like a nursing cap.

My assignments included helping on a medical and surgical floor, working in Radiology, and manning the information desk in the hospital lobby. I visited with the patients while providing water, cards, flowers, newspapers, and linen. I also ran errands throughout the hospital, helped transport patients on gurneys or wheelchairs, and directed visitors to patient rooms or hospital departments. I recall running an errand to the operating room, and although I couldn't proceed beyond the entry doors, I was thrilled just to be up there with my little piece of equipment. This valuable experience allowed me to visit with the nurses and observe firsthand their roles and responsibilities. And I LOVED it.

Working as a Nursing Assistant in 1966 at Mason District Hospital, Havana, Illinois, afforded me several interesting experiences. Caring for actual patients, I learned to feed, bathe, turn, provide bedpans, make beds, and transport patients. After expressing my interest in working in surgery, I was invited to visit the operating room to see it first-hand. I wasn't allowed to observe an operation, but just seeing the suite was rewarding. I also had my first experience with death when one of my patients died.

The summer following my junior year in high school, I learned that one could "hand instruments to the doctor" in the operating room. Thinking this would be a great summer job and ignorant of the complexities the role entailed, I made an appointment to speak with someone at Methodist Hospital School of Nursing in Peoria, where I expressed my interest in pursuing this job. Knowing now the complexity and skill required by the Surgical Technologist, I laugh to think of doing this for a summer job. However, the Lord uses people and circumstances to guide and direct us as He works out His plan for us. Such was the case with this meeting. After relaying my desire to work as a Surgical Technologist as a summer job, no less, the director of the school explained that this was more involved than a summer job. She then encouraged me to pursue a career in nursing rather than limiting myself to the technical aspect of passing instruments. She presented the education required and reviewed the benefits of pursuing a Baccalaureate Degree in Nursing. A very confident and straightforward woman, she encouraged me and validated the desire to pursue my nursing dreams.

My interest in a nursing career morphed into a curiosity regarding anesthesia. After writing a high school term paper regarding a career as an Anesthetist, I determined this would be my path. However, God had other plans for me. I maintained this goal until I was accepted into Anesthesia school two years into my career. After observing the significant time commitment, long hours, and frequent on-call obligations, I decided to withdraw my application from the school and close that door. I recall feeling sad as I informed the director of my decision to withdraw my application, and I was to question that decision for years. The passage of time often brings clarity, and as the years passed and my career progressed to the administrative track, I realized I was in the right place. Because I loved what I was doing, any remaining regrets or second-guessing vanished.

# 3

## Nursing Education Begins

*Joshua 1:9 Be strong and courageous. Do not be frightened, and do not be dismayed, for the Lord your God is with you wherever you go.*

Having fulfilled the necessary math, biology, chemistry, and anatomy courses in high school, it was time to move on to nursing school. As someone for whom math is not a strong suit, I was grateful to complete basic Algebra and Geometry classes without progressing to the more advanced courses. When I later discovered that math would become integral to my career, I wished I had paid better attention and worked harder to understand it. Interestingly, because of an excellent English teacher, I briefly considered following in her footsteps and teaching English. However, the inner drive returned, drawing me back to Nursing - I was called.

In 1968, there were basically two school choices – obtain a diploma in nursing from a three-year hospital-sponsored program or attend a university and obtain a Bachelor of Science in Nursing (BSN). I perceived that the BSN would be beneficial if I wished to pursue a supervisory role. While two-year Associate Degree programs were an option, I wasn't aware of any schools. I only considered a four-year college degree or a diploma school.

Nursing Explorer website states, "Diploma programs are the oldest and most traditional form of nursing education in the United States," having started in the 1870s in several major U.S. cities (Author Unknown, Nursing Explorer, 2012). They were usually three-year programs based in a hospital setting, whose popularity spread rapidly across the country. Diploma nursing schools were originally considered a source of unpaid hospital labor, with students working 12 hours a day or longer. Education at a diploma school was very hands-on as students assumed responsibility for the total care of their patients. With its emphasis on clinical experience and direct patient care, the diploma schools provide more clinical instruction than any other nursing program, which many students find appealing (Author Unknown, Nursing Explorer, 2012).

Diploma schools reached their peak of 1,300 schools nationwide in the 1950s and 1960s, with graduates receiving a diploma rather than a college degree. Although similar to the Associate's Degree in Nursing (ADN) programs, the diploma program still offers the highest number of clinical hours, allowing graduates to reach clinical competence rapidly. Fewer than 100 diploma nursing schools remain in the United States (Author Unknown, Nursing Explorer, 2012).

As many can attest, applying to and choosing a school of higher learning can be daunting and intimidating. Surprisingly, I didn't initially apply to hospital-based diploma nursing programs but to colleges and universities. I was accepted into the liberal arts program at Northern Illinois University in DeKalb, Illinois. A high school friend, already a student there, invited me to spend the weekend with her. I eagerly anticipated the weekend on what I thought would be my future campus. While I enjoyed spending time with her, meeting her friends, staying in the dorm, and touring the campus, my enthusiasm for attending there waned. However, I moved forward and applied to their College of Nursing. I was informed of the requirement to complete a year of liberal arts courses, at which time I could submit my application to the school of nursing. Concerned that my acceptance into the Nursing Program could be delayed or possibly not even happen, I pursued other educational opportunities.

Applications to numerous Illinois diploma schools of nursing ensued – Passavant in Jacksonville, Methodist and St. Francis Schools of Nursing in Peoria, Graham Hospital in Canton (still in existence), and Mennonite in Bloomington. I felt drawn to Mennonite.

With Mennonite's application process looking promising, my parents and I visited the school and met with Dr. Jacqueline Kinder, the program Director. I was impressed with this very kind, educated, articulate woman of faith. I recall sitting in her office as she reviewed the program with our family and answered our questions. Her friendly smile and kind demeanor put me at ease. Through the years, I deeply respected her as a person and a leader because her personal and professional life aligned with her faith in Christ.

I went through the admission process, and upon being accepted into Mennonite's program, I began preparing for my next life journey. There were many unknowns – who would be my roommate, would we get along, would I make friends with whom I could be as close as my high school friends, would I enjoy nursing as much as I thought I would, could I do it? Could I pass college Chemistry? Could I deal with other people's bodily functions? Would I fit in? Would this conservative environment be too restricting? Yikes.

Mennonite was a small Christian school that ascribed to Biblical principles. Although I was not yet a Christian, their beliefs felt comfortable and compatible with my Methodist upbringing. It was close to home yet far enough away to gain some independence, and I was familiar with the Bloomington-Normal area. Its affiliation with Illinois State University (ISU) provided a taste of college life.

Our classes at ISU established a foundation in liberal arts and science. We earned 30 college credits for coursework in English, Nutrition, Chemistry, Microbiology, two semesters of Anatomy and Physiology, Child Development, Psychology, Political Science, English Literature, and Sociology. After completing additional classes, I graduated with 36 college credit hours. These course credits proved beneficial in later years when I obtained my Undergraduate and Graduate degrees. I experienced college life by spending most weekends with one of my high school friends who attended Illinois State University.

Having enjoyed a wonderful grade school, junior high, and high school experience, I was blessed with a group of close friends (who remain friends to this day). We formed strong bonds and had a lot of fun together. While excited to finally pursue my lifelong dream of nursing, it was hard to think of leaving home and friends. The thought of cultivating new relationships with new experiences and challenges was daunting for this 18-year-old.

High school graduation came and went, and I said goodbye to people with whom I had been friends since kindergarten. Leaving these people was difficult because I was liked and accepted, and I knew the ropes, so to speak. Moving into the unknown was unsettling.

I received luggage for my high school graduation – evidence I was headed somewhere. With the passing of summer, preparations for school were in full swing. Unlike today's college-bound students, we didn't spend hundreds of dollars on dorm necessities at Walmart, Kohl's, or Target. Those stores did not even exist. The school provided bedding and towels which were exchanged weekly. Curtains were already on the windows. We purchased a serviceable olive-green twin bedspread, a reading lamp, an alarm clock, a yellow pillow with armrests for sitting up in bed, and some miscellaneous items.

Given the school's religious affiliation with the Mennonite Church, students were expected to be of high moral character, affiliated with a church, and refrain from tobacco or alcohol use. Notice that illegal drug use was not mentioned because it wasn't considered an issue at that time. The Mennonite Hospital School of Nursing 1970 handbook provides a concise historical background of the school and is presented in its entirety as follows:

Mennonite Hospital is a general hospital under the direction and control of the Mennonite Hospital Association, which is composed of members of some 40 Mennonite Churches in Central Illinois. Dedicated in 1919, the hospital had expanded by 1959 to provide 130 acute beds and 23 bassinets.

Another expansion project, which began in the fall of 1967, will double the hospital's capacity. At the completion of the project, the hospital will provide 114 acute beds, 5 intensive care beds, 50 rehabilitation beds, 20 self-care beds, and 80 extended-care beds.

Mennonite Hospital, in conjunction with the Gailey Eye Clinic, sponsors an Eye Bank, and one nursing unit provides specialized care for patients recuperating from eye surgery.

In addition to the School of Nursing, the hospital offers education programs for Medical Technologists and X-Ray Technologists.

The School of Nursing was established in 1919 to implement the hospital's two-fold purpose: to provide a Christian ministry of healing to the sick and injured and to provide instruction for qualified persons who desired to become nurses. The first class graduated in 1922.

The present four-story building which houses the School of Nursing and residence unit was dedicated in 1946 as Troyer Memorial Nurses' Home, in memory of the Rev. Emmanuel Troyer, who served as president of the Board of Trustees from the beginning of the work until his death in 1942. The building stands directly east of the hospital, on East Street, and is connected with the hospital by an underground concourse (Mennonite Hospital School of Nursing Catalog 1967-68, p. 3).

The 1970 handbook provided the following learning objectives for our three-year educational pursuit:

- To acquire a body of knowledge, skills, and attitudes through which she develops herself, with proper guidance, into an active member of the health team.
- To develop through a variety of structured learning experiences the ability to plan and give total nursing care.
- To develop communication skills that enable her to relate effectively to the patient and his family, to the members

of the health team, and to others with whom she comes in contact.
- To develop the ability to analyze nursing problems and to use sound judgment in making decisions.
- To qualify for a beginning staff position and to recognize the need and responsibility for continued growth (Hoover and Kapp, 1985, p 3).

These objectives reveal that nursing was predominantly a female profession. The lack of reference to male students, evidenced by the omission of male pronouns, assumes that students will be female. Upon checking Mennonite's graduating classes from 1950 to 1985, I found the first male graduate in 1964. One male graduated in the classes of 1967 and 1973. In 1981 there were three, and in 1982 and 1983, there were two male graduates each year.

About a month before leaving for school, I received a letter from someone I had never met. She introduced herself and said she would be my "big sis" at school. I was overjoyed because, as an only child, I had never enjoyed a sisterly bond. The letter was filled with kindness as she assured me that she would help me adjust to the school. She was confident that I would be happy there and that we would be great friends. She was a lifeline to this new place and life. I was impressed that she took the time to send that letter, plus several more as we corresponded throughout the summer. Because email and social media did not exist, we had no electronic communication, and long-distance phone calls incurred a fee. We could not "friend" each other on Facebook because it was nonexistent. The U.S. Postal Service provided our preferred means of communication until we met in person.

One by one, my hometown friends left for school, jobs, or military service around the same time I did. The day before I left, while my mother was working, my friend Cynthia and I were actively preparing to leave for college. I included a picture of us "packing and organizing" my things before we started on hers. And we wondered why our parents were concerned.

Throughout the preparations, my parents refrained from saying much, but as their only child, my departure must have been difficult for them. The house would be quieter without my friends bouncing in and out of our back door. Would they miss the door slamming behind me as I took off to socialize with my friends? As I was to learn many years later, my grandparents were an integral part of my educational opportunities. And although I was never actually told, I know my parents and grandparents prayed for me. I was excited to realize that my lifelong dream of becoming a nurse could be a reality, but in my heart, I knew it could never be the same. And as I would later learn – once I left my little hometown, I left for good. I returned for visits, but I never lived there again.

Sometimes, we vividly recall the intricate details of significant events just as we experienced them. Such was my departure from home. It was a warm, sunny August Saturday when my scant worldly belongings, suitcases, and a few boxes were loaded into my dad's 1964 green Ford Fairlane. Resolute with leaving, I closed the kitchen door behind me and hopped into the backseat for the drive out of town and away from home. I recall pondering the familiarity of where I grew up, having spent so many happy days as a child and teenager. Then, unexpectedly, my nose began to bleed, and we had to return home to get it stopped. Oh boy- I just experienced the feeling of leaving, and now I have returned home for a repeat exit. Once the nosebleed stopped, however, I had little time to think about leaving again because we needed to arrive at the school's welcome assembly on time.

I was understandably nervous as we arrived at the dorm, parked the car, and proceeded to the entrance. I was delighted to see a very lovely girl waiting on the steps. She said, "Are you Ila?" When I replied that I was, she introduced herself and said she would be my "big sis". For months, my fellow freshman classmates remarked how lucky I was to have her as my "big sis". She was a valued and treasured lifeline. Her demeanor was kind and enthusiastic as she introduced herself to my parents and escorted us to the welcoming assembly. I have learned through the years that although I was not yet a Christian, God faithfully brought people into my life to guide, support, comfort, and love me. She was one of those people

Our freshman class was comprised of girls, except for one man. My dad was intrigued that a man would choose a nursing career because, in 1968, men rarely pursued a career in nursing. In fact, in 1968, only a handful of professions were considered suitable for women. These professions included teacher, beautician, secretary, stewardess (now called flight attendant), and nurse. Women gravitated toward nursing, and men gravitated toward the physician role. It was common for women to be homemakers and remain at home to raise their families and care for the house while the men served as breadwinners. It was not uncommon for girls to be married right out of high school and start a family shortly after.

The faculty, new students, families, and returning students assembled in the auditorium on the dorm's lower level. We were welcomed by the director and introduced to the faculty. We then went around the room and introduced ourselves. I was grateful for the school's obvious Christian mission and influence and felt confident I had chosen the correct place. Looking back, I am grateful that the parents were integrated into this welcome assembly. It gave everyone a chance to see where their daughters and sons would reside, be educated, and with whom they would be spending their time.

Following the assembly, we proceeded to our assigned dorm room to meet our new roommates, unpack, get settled, and say goodbye to our parents. The luggage and a few boxes holding all of my earthly belongings were retrieved from my dad's car. Unloading required little time and effort because I did not have a carload of items. School supplies, articles for the dorm room, toiletries, clothing, and a few pictures were arranged in their appropriate places. Because two of my grandchildren are Korean adoptees, I now find it interesting that my first roommate was a Korean adoptee. My parents had the opportunity to meet her and her mother as we arranged our new living space and settled in. We made the beds, unpacked our suitcases, and set our meager belongings around that stark room. I am certain it put my parents at ease to meet the person with whom I would be living and get acquainted with her mother.

Our family refrained from physical expressions of affection, so when it came time for my parents to leave, I simply walked them out and told them goodbye. I recall feeling quite alone standing there and watching them drive away. The unknown can be very unsettling, and at 18, three years seemed like a long time.

Because it was Saturday, we had the remainder of that day and Sunday before classes began. My roommate and I shared information about ourselves to get acquainted.

We discussed our families, friends, town, and activities we enjoyed as we walked around Bloomington. Although a very pleasant girl, it was soon obvious that her interest in a nursing career was waning as she enjoyed a robust social life, rarely studied, and ultimately dropped out after her first semester.

Another student and I quickly developed a friendship and became roommates second semester, remaining roommates through our junior year. Her personality, sense of humor, and antics made rooming with her delightful. We were compatible and had great times as our friendship grew and blossomed. Her home was in Florida, where she was valedictorian of her high school graduating class. She was the oldest of ten children, making our childhoods vastly different. Stories of her and her siblings kept me entertained. She said her mother used to post signs around the house, and I still recall finding the "eat it now or hide it" signage amusing.

Monday morning dawned bright and sunny, our first day as student nurses! The initial days were spent in orientation before classes began at Illinois State University (ISU) and Mennonite. The student nurses did not drive to ISU, nor did we walk. The humility of all humility – the mode of transportation awaiting us was an old school bus painted turquoise blue and named Virgil. Make no mistake, it was turquoise blue. And it was old! This spectacle transported us to ISU for our classes there. I suspect that the bus was a gift to the school because surely, they had not spent money on it. We bounced along through the streets of Bloomington and Normal wending our way to the university. Hitting a pothole would send us rocketing out of our seats. We endured bitter cold in the winter and hot air in the summer with a barely functioning heater and, of course, no air conditioning. We had to laugh because it was just too embarrassing. And all of the ISU students knew who we were when that goofy ancient relic of a bus pulled into campus – the nurses had arrived! While conducting my research about Mennonite and the school's history, I searched in vain for a picture of "Virgil". However, it is fairly easy to compile a mental picture.

Fortunately, Mennonite school administrators had the foresight to recognize that nursing's future resided in the baccalaureate-prepared nurse. Most diploma programs provided all courses at the school, where students completed Anatomy and Physiology, Microbiology, Chemistry, etc., without the benefit of accumulating college credits. If those students decided to pursue a baccalaureate degree following graduation from the diploma school, they were forced to repeat previously completed courses. As a bonus, I met my husband at ISU while attending summer school there. The book's photo section includes a picture of Terry and me taken in 2018, seated on the "Those Who Fell in Love at ISU" bench on the ISU campus.

**Dorm Life**

The student dorm was attached to the hospital via a tunnel, allowing us direct access to the hospital without going outside. The hospital was located on the main thoroughfare through Bloomington/Normal, and the dorm was directly behind the hospital on a quiet residential street.

The dorm was a neat but modest brick residence hall of four floors. My first room was on the fourth floor, and we resided on the third floor during our junior year. Stairs were the mode of moving from floor to floor. I do not recall having an elevator. The first floor housed the library and an auditorium for chapel, social gatherings, and some classes. The kitchen, laundry facilities, and the tunnel entrance to the hospital were also contained on the first floor. Our classroom and clinical practice areas were located in a large room adjacent to the tunnel. The walls were painted mint green, and the floors were dark green and black tile. Each floor had one bathroom with multiple wooden stalls, older porcelain sinks, and individual showers with curtains. Only single female students were allowed to reside in the dorm. Married or male students were housed off-campus. Students living in the Bloomington-Normal area could reside at home, although the local resident students I knew preferred staying in the dorm.

Lack of air-conditioning necessitated wide open windows and portable fans whirring at high speed in warm weather. Ceiling fans did not exist except in department stores. The serviceable maple (maybe pine?) furniture consisted of two single beds, two dressers, and a shared desk. Two small closets rounded out our minimal storage. The uncomfortable mattresses caused many of us to suffer from backaches. We kept Gerald, the maintenance man, busy placing plywood between the springs and the mattress to improve support. Anytime maintenance was required, we would hear a loud announcement, "Man on the floor," prompting us to scurry to our rooms before they entered the hallway.

Each floor was equipped with one rotary phone housed in a small phone booth shared by everyone on that floor. When the phone rang, whoever was near would answer it and shout down the hall to summon the intended recipient. We usually knew who was present on the floor, so finding the person was rarely a problem. If we were absent when we received a call, we found a note with a message taped to our door when we returned. Long-distance calls were made via the operator collect to the intended recipient, usually our parents. Cell phones would have been futuristic, and we could not have imagined such indulgences.

If we had a visitor, the housemother notified us by calling our name via our floor intercom, and when we answered, we were informed that we had a visitor in the lobby. No visitor was allowed on the floors unless accompanied by one of us. Boyfriends were never allowed on the dorm residential floors.

A stairway led from the fourth floor to the roof, where we sunbathed in warmer weather. A large living room adjacent to the entrance provided a gathering area for family or other visitors. Although we were all of legal age at 18 and older, we had a 10 PM curfew on weeknights and midnight on weekends, and we were required to sign in and out of the dorm. Very few of the women drank alcohol, but those who did realized that arriving back at the dorm inebriated risked unpleasant consequences. Two of the students made the mistake of hiding liquor in their room and were summarily dismissed from the program. Men in the dorm? Unthinkable and didn't happen.

We had 24-hour supervision from two resident housemothers who lived on the third and fourth floors and enjoyed a private bathroom in their little apartments. They staffed the front desk morning, noon, and night until curfew to make sure we followed the rules. Other women filled in at the front desk, but only two lived there. Men were NEVER allowed on the residential floors for social visits. To my knowledge, no one ever snuck someone in.

Our meals were eaten in the hospital cafeteria located off the tunnel. I recall the food was not terrible. Meals were of the traditional content of that time, consisting of meat, potatoes, vegetables, rolls, salad, and dessert. Pizza and chicken tenders were not among the offerings. Thankfully, our high activity level prevented much weight gain from that calorie-packed menu laden with sugar, carbohydrates, and fat. Hospital renovation provided a new and much larger cafeteria for our junior and senior years. Snacks and personal food could be labeled and stored in the lounge refrigerators on each floor. Microwaves became popular in the 1970s but were unavailable to Mennonite nursing students from 1968 to 1971. Therefore, we prepared food via a stovetop, oven, or the ever-popular hot plate. I remember the smell of burned Campbell's bean with bacon soup wafting from the room of two of my friends when they left it on the hot plate a little too long. Bean with bacon soup seemed to be a staple meal for us.

The front stairs to the dorm entrance were the scene of many hellos and goodbyes from family, boyfriends, and friends. If those steps could talk, they would have revealed professions of love, break-ups, happy greetings, many kisses and hugs, and merry skipping footsteps down to greet someone special. I returned to the site of the hospital and dorm when I researched this book. The hospital is gone and many of the dorm's windows are boarded up. Even looking at the wreckage of what was once my student home, I was drawn to those steps and flooded with many memories of events there.

Illinois Wesleyan Theta Chi fraternity was across the street from the hospital, with Illinois Wesleyan University just a few short blocks away. Because we were tucked away, we didn't draw much attention from the fraternity gentlemen or any other gentlemen for that matter. I occasionally used Illinois Wesleyan's library to study. I enjoyed a break from Mennonite studying in a different surrounding than the dorm, mingling with other college students.

The second floor served as the main entrance with the housemother's desk, mailboxes, a couple of classrooms, the school nurse's office, and a few dorm rooms. The isolation "sick" room was located on that floor, across the hall from the school nurse's office and the housemother's desk. If deemed contagious, you were assigned to the sick room without access to television or radio, with nothing but a bed and other sparse furniture present.

I experienced the misfortune of contracting the Hong Kong flu at Christmastime in 1968. Rather than sending me home because it was close to Christmas break, I was sequestered alone in the isolation room. My friends waved to me through the door. One day (yes, I was there for days) the school nurse came for me, instructed me to put on a robe, and marched me through the tunnel, passed the gawking eyes of the hospital staff, and into the emergency room where the school physician was waiting for me with a shot of penicillin. I was then returned to the isolation room and put back to bed. All meals were brought to me. I do not recall if I had anything to read, but I remember being very sick with a fever and a bad cough. One evening, I snuck out of the room, called my dad at home, and asked if he would come and get me. Somehow, the school nurse got wind of it, contacted my parents, and I was allowed to go home. I am uncertain if my parents were ever informed that I was sick before I called them. I recovered in time to enjoy Christmas. I avoided the misfortune of spending time in the isolation room again. It was enough of a deterrent that no one would ever fake an illness.

Without the benefit of owning a car, transportation was provided by city bus, taxi, or walking. There were no cell phones and therefore no access to help should trouble arise. This was the norm, and we did not think twice about it. I would often hop on the city bus on Friday afternoon heading to ISU, then sometimes walk back carrying my overnight bag on my return trip on Sunday because the buses did not run on Sunday.

I frequently received mail. Because long-distance calls incurred a fee, I wrote letters to my parents and grandparents. My grandmother faithfully wrote weekly letters to me. I had to call my parents collect to talk to them. Calls were infrequent because collect calls were even more expensive than direct dial long-distance calls. Although Terry and I spent time together, we also exchanged letters via mail. Looking back, I have fond memories of receiving "love" letters from him, even though he was only a few miles away.

Saturday, November 9, 1968, offered a rare but significant seismic event in central Illinois. I was awakened around 11 AM (yes, I was still asleep at 11 AM) to my little dorm bed violently shaking and slowly working its way across the room. Still half asleep, I thought my roommate was shaking my bed, and I wondered why she would do such a thing. Realizing my roommate was not even in the room, I could not imagine what was happening. Wikipedia describes the event as the "largest recorded earthquake in the state of Illinois, measuring 5.3 on the Richter scale," and it was felt over a large area of the Midwest (Wikipedia contributors, 2024). Although there were no fatalities, some areas sustained significant structural damage.

## Curriculum

Our curriculum and clinical experiences from 1968 to 1971 differ from today's students' experiences. I located our curriculum in the handbook, which consisted of the following:

| | | |
|---|---|---|
| Nutrition 106 | 2 Semester Hours | ISU |
| Chemistry 104 | 3 Semester Hours | ISU |
| Religion in Nursing 205 | 2 Term Hours | Mennonite |
| Pharmacology | | Mennonite |
| Medical Terminology | | Mennonite |
| Language and Composition 101 | 3 Semester Hours | ISU |
| Foundations in Nursing 101 | 4 Semester Hours | Mennonite |
| Adult Nursing 101 | 6 Semester Hours | Mennonite |
| Adult Nursing 201, 202 | 10 Term Hours | Mennonite |
| Advanced Surgical Nursing 203 | 10 Term Hrs | Mennonite |
| Maternal and Infant Nursing 204 | 10 Term Hrs | Mennonite |
| Adult Nursing 301 | 10 Term Hours | Mennonite |
| Adult Nursing 302 | 8 Term Hours | Mennonite |
| Adult Nursing 303 | 6 Term Hours | Mennonite |
| Foundations of Nursing 301. | 2 Term Hours | Mennonite |
| Pediatric Nursing | 8 Term Hours | Varied |
| Psychiatric Nursing | 15 Term Hours | Peoria State Hospital |
| | | Brokaw Hospital |

(Hoover and Kapp, 1985)

Because this list was gleaned from the student catalog, I am uncertain why it doesn't include all of the required ISU courses, as we also enrolled in Psychology, two semesters of Anatomy and Physiology with laboratory experience, and Child Development. The required courses in Pharmacology and Medical Terminology are also omitted from this list.

As previously mentioned, the focus of a diploma school was developing clinical skills and nursing judgment. I will always maintain that diploma school graduates possess the strongest clinical (AKA nursing) skills because of the program's clinical emphasis. We worked all shifts, including nights, during our education. As evidenced by the curriculum, we enjoyed some liberal arts classes, but the major focus was the development of nursing and clinical skills. In addition, our school year was ten months long, beginning mid-August until mid to late June. Christmas break was two weeks, Easter break was a week, and we only enjoyed semester break freshman year.

Despite the "Virgil" humiliation, I enjoyed attending college, especially Anatomy and Physiology classes. However, I found the laboratory experience challenging. The lab was taught by a graduate student and consisted of dissecting former living things like sharks, piglets, and frogs to identify muscles and nerves. Tuesday and Thursday evenings found us seated on stools, hovering over our "project" with surgical instruments in hand, dissecting and locating animal or fish body parts. The smell of formaldehyde permeated the room. To test our knowledge, exams consisted of "stations" containing animals in various stages of dissection. A pin marked the body part we were to identify on the exam. We would then enter the name of the muscle or nerve in front of us.

We memorized every bone in the body, the muscles, and the cranial nerves. Point to a bone on a skeleton, and we could name it. Cranial nerves were learned using the mnemonic "On Old Olympus's Towering Top, a Finn and German viewed some Hops". This helped us remember the

Olfactory, Optic, Oculomotor, Trochlear, Trigeminal, Abducens, Facial, Vestibulocochlear, Glossopharyngeal, Vagus, Accessory, and Hypoglossal nerves. We recited those nerves while walking through the halls, riding on the bus, or sitting in our rooms. Pointing to our skeletal structure while identifying our bones helped hard-wire the names of all 206 bones in the human body. When I started working in the operating room, I was required to know all of those body parts.

As someone not blessed with stellar math skills, I struggled mightily with Chemistry and its algebraic chemical equations. Studying the coursework was frustrating because I did not understand what I was reading. The professor offered her help, and I passed the course. (I did not understand Algebra until I enrolled in an introductory Algebra class at 37 years of age in preparation for returning to school for my BSN.)

Lest one conclude it was all books and studying, take heart because we managed some school/life balance. Composition and Language (i.e., English) class ended at 4 PM on Monday and Wednesday afternoons. Because many of us were fans of the popular soap opera Dark Shadows, we were tempted to skip the class, hop on the city bus, and return to the dorm to catch the 3 PM episode. Occasionally, we yielded to that temptation. On those days, we could be found huddled around the little black and white TV in the 4th-floor lounge, watching the vampire Barnabus Collins attempt to claim his next victim. Our English grade, fortunately, did not suffer due to our dalliance.

Contrast my curriculum with the current traditional BSN track at Mennonite College of Nursing at Illinois State University. The plan of study from the traditional four-year

BSN College of Nursing website presents the following course requirements:

**Freshman Year**

| | | |
|---|---|---|
| English 101 | Composition as Critical Inquiry | 3 Semester Hours (SH) |
| HSC 105 | Medical Terminology | 3 SH |
| Psy 110 | Fundamentals of Psychology | 3 SH |
| Com 110 | Communication as Critical Inquiry | 3 SH |
| BSC | Microbiology and Society | 4 SH |
| CHE 110/112 | Chemistry | 4 SH |
| GE | Math | 4 SH |
| GE | General Education | |

**Sophomore Year**

| | | |
|---|---|---|
| FCS 102 | Fundamentals of Human Nutrition | 3 SH |
| BSC 181 | Human Physiology and Anatomy | 4 SH |
| BSC 182 | Human Physiology and Anatomy | 4 SH |
| ECO 138 | Statistics | 3 SH |
| Nurs 224 | Contemporary Professional Nursing | 1 SH |
| Nurs 237 | Cultural and Spiritual Dimensions of Healthcare | 1 SH |
| PSY 213 | Lifespan Development | 3 SH |

**Junior Year**

| | | |
|---|---|---|
| Nsg 222 | Psychomotor Skills for Nursing | 3 SH |
| Nsg 239 | Pathophysiology and Pharmacotherapeutics in Nursing | 3 SH |
| Nsg 339 | Pathophysiology and Pharmacotherapeutics in Nursing | 3 SH |
| Nsg 225 | Health Assessment of the Adult | 4 SH |

| | | |
|---|---|---|
| Nsg 229 | Adult Nursing | 6 SH |
| Nsg 316 | Maternal Infant Nursing | 4 SH |
| Nsg 231 | Adult Nursing | 7 SH |
| Nsg 336 | Research and Theory for Evidenced-Based Practice | 3 SH |

**Senior Year**

| | | |
|---|---|---|
| Nsg 317 | Nursing Care of Children | 4 SH |
| Nsg 314 | Psychiatric and Mental Health Nursing | 6 SH |
| Nsg 329 | Public Health Nursing | 5 SH |
| Nsg 325 | Adult Nursing III | 7 SH |
| Nsg 327 | Leadership Dimensions in Nursing | 6 SH |
| Nsg 326 | Gerontological Nursing | 2 SH |

(Mennonite Plan of Study, 2024)

    Current nursing education enjoys a broader scope encompassing liberal arts, leadership, research, community, all stages of development, and the world. Twenty-first-century nursing students replicate actual patient scenarios through high-tech, state-of-the-art simulation labs with sophisticated "patients" that reflect a precise response to illness and treatment. Our simulation experience included practicing on the mannequin patient "Mrs. Chase", actual patients, and often classmates. In the 2023-2024 issue of The Flame, Mennonite announced the opening of its new state-of-the-art simulation center that boasts a "60-seat classroom, a technology room for virtual reality programming, three fully immersive technology rooms, a fully functioning four-bed hospital unit, hospital simulation space, undergraduate skills and health assessment labs, faculty offices, conference and study areas" (The Flame 2023-2024, p. 5).

# Chapel

Attending a Christian school meant we were required to participate in the weekly chapel service held in the first-floor school auditorium. Arranging the chairs in rows gave the room a "churchy" feel. The beautiful music and time away from classes provided a nice respite from our school responsibilities. Someone played the piano as our voices harmonized beautiful hymns such as Day by Day and With Each Passing Moment, I Know Whom I Have Believed, and others. A speaker provided a short devotional, and we ended the service with a prayer. Speakers might be local pastors, the hospital chaplain, former students, nursing faculty, or someone sharing an inspirational story. Sometimes, we had special music – a duet, trio, or sextet. I occasionally participated in the sextet or choir. I remember our school director and her husband sang, her beautiful alto voice blending with his as they honored God with song.

*Day by Day and With Each Passing Moment*

*Day by day and with each passing moment,*
*Strength I find to meet my trials here*
*Trusting in my Father's wise bestowment,*
*I've no cause for worry or for fear.*
*He whose heart is kind beyond all measure*
*Gives unto each day what He deems best-*
*Lovingly, it's part of pain and pleasure,*
*Mingling toil with peace and rest.*

*Every day, the Lord Himself is near me*
*With a special mercy for each hour;*
*All my cares He fain would bear and cheer me,*
*He whose name is Counselor and Power.*

*The protection of His child and treasure*
*Is a charge that on Himself He laid;*
*As thy days, thy strength shall be in measure*
*This the pledge to me He made.*

*Help me then in every tribulation*
*so to trust Thy promises, O Lord,*
*that I lose not faith's sweet consolation*
*offered me within Thy holy word.*
*Help me Lord, when toil and trouble meeting,*
*e'er to take, as from a father's hand,*
*one by one, the days, the moments fleeting,*
*'til I reach the promised land.*              *(Berg, 1865)*

<u>I Know Whom I Have Believed</u>

*I know not why God's wondrous grace*
*To me He hath made known,*
*Nor why, unworthy, Christ in love*
*Redeemed me for His own*

*I know not when my Lord may come,*
*At night, or noonday fair,*
*Nor if I walk the vale with Him,*
*Or meet Him in the air.*
*(Chorus:)*
*But I know whom I have believed,*
*And am persuaded that He is able*
*To keep that which I've committed*
*Unto Him against that day.*              *(Whittle, 1883)*

I attended my hometown's Methodist church from infancy. My father was the organist, my mother and grandmother taught Sunday school, and I actively participated in the music program. Therefore, I had heard about Jesus from my earliest childhood. I knew about his birth, death on the cross, and His resurrection from the dead. However, I had never personally embraced Jesus' gift of salvation. I had never truly accepted it as something He did for *me*. Avoiding any reflection on my own sin, I had never considered His death and resurrection in a deeply personal way. It was not due to never hearing the plan of salvation, I had just never confessed my sins, asked God to forgive me, and accepted Christ's atoning death and resurrection as the only way to heaven.

During one of our weekly chapel services, a lady from a local church shared the importance of accepting Christ as one's personal Savior. Her presentation and delivery of the message resonated with me, and I knew it was time to make a life-changing decision for Christ. She invited us to call her if we wanted to discuss what she had said. After contacting her, she picked me up at the nurse's dorm and took me to the Steak 'n Shake where she explained the gospel message. I understood that although I had attended church my entire life, I needed to make this very personal decision. I acknowledged that Jesus died on the cross to forgive MY sins, and I accepted Him as my Savior in April of my freshman year.

# 4

## Freshman Year 1968-1969

*Psalm 32: 8, 9 I will instruct you and teach you in the way you should go; I will counsel you with my eye upon you.*

When my nursing journey began, nursing education was called Nurse's Training, perhaps because we were "trained" to be clinically strong. Developing impeccable clinical skills and sound nursing judgment was the foundation of our educational process. One of my physician colleagues used to ask me if I was educated or trained. He implied that animals are trained, but nurses are educated. Reflecting on that question, I concluded that nurses are both educated and trained. For me, the education component came in numerous forms – college classes, nursing textbooks, lectures, anecdotal information received from senior colleagues and physicians, and my independent reading and research. However, training is part of the nurse's comprehensive education. We are educated regarding the principles of critical thinking, but are trained to carry them out. Consider that we are educated regarding the principles and reasons for intravenous (IV) therapy but are trained to insert an IV, calculate the drip, assess the patient's response to the treatment, and titrate the medication based on physician orders. Trained to administer medication and educated regarding the purpose and actions of each one.

In the early fall of 1968, during our freshman year, we formally dedicated our lives to nursing during a ceremony at Wesley United Methodist Church in Bloomington, Illinois. Our dedication to nursing was similar to a pinning, capping, stethoscope, or white coat ceremony. Our class of student nurses processed in as the organist played Trumpet Voluntary on the majestic pipe organ. My parents, grandparents, and the parents of two high school friends honored me with their attendance. I was filled with pride and close to tears as I walked the long aisle with my classmates. Our school choir sang a special number in beautiful harmony. Each freshman class member received a small white Nightingale lamp with a single candle lit by the school director. The Nightingale pledge, composed in 1893, was recited from memory and in unison. As the pledge indicates, nurses were responsible and subservient to the physician.

I solemnly pledge myself before God and in the presence of this assembly, to pass my life in purity and to practice my profession faithfully. I will abstain from whatever is deleterious and mischievous, and will not take or knowingly administer any harmful drug. I will do all in my power to maintain and elevate the standard of my profession and will hold in confidence all personal matters committed to my keeping and all family affairs coming to my knowledge in the practice of my calling. With loyalty will I endeavor to aid the physician in his work, and devote myself to the welfare of those committed to my care (Vanderbilt School of Nursing, 2010).

I kept that lamp for many years, but it finally disappeared during one of our moves. The photo section contains pictures of the program and a lamp.

Our first introduction to actual nursing occurred in the Fundamentals of Nursing class, where we learned basic patient care. Our instructor was a stickler for practicing "by the book" with no deviation. She set high expectations for a professional nursing career in our dress, actions, and interactions with physicians, staff, and patients. It was never acceptable to address a physician by his/her first name. I know she successfully drilled this into me because I have always found it difficult to address a physician by his or her first name. One physician colleague and friend once remarked that he had a first name to which I replied, "Yes, and your first name is Doctor".

Basic nursing care encompasses taking vital signs, turning a patient, feeding a patient, giving a bed bath, placing and removing a bedpan, fundamentals of charting nurses' notes, chart components, and helping the patient transfer to a chair and ambulate. Vital signs included taking the temperature, palpating the pulse, observing respirations, and taking the patient's blood pressure. These numbers were documented by hand on the assignment sheet and entered manually into the TPR (temperature, pulse, respiration) graph. As students, we entered these numbers ourselves. Otherwise, the nursing staff documented the results for the Unit Clerk to record in the patient's graph. Electronic charting would not become a reality for decades, so black and red ink pens were staples. Black ink was used to document in the patient's chart, and red ink was used if a documentation error occurred. Some organizations charted the PM or night shift nurse's notes with red ink. Any error required that a single line be drawn through the error in red ink, the error was dated, and our initials were inserted to indicate who documented the error. One wanted to avoid making numerous errors because that red ink stood out.

We were taught to make a hospital bed with or without a patient occupying it. We were expected to tuck a tight draw sheet around the bottom sheet and produce neat, precise hospital corners. The bottom sheet was not fitted, so the draw sheet served as an anchor to keep that sheet in place and to turn the patient when necessary for repositioning or transfer. To this day, I cannot make a bed without hospital corners, and I have been known to rip out hotel sheets to create them. Through the years, I have found that many nursing colleagues share the same obsession with bed-making. When making our bed, my husband places the fitted sheet, but when it comes to the top sheet, he says that's above his pay grade.

State-of-the-art simulation labs with sophisticated mannequins capable of replicating real medical scenarios did not yet exist. Our simulation was conducted on Mrs. Chase, a life-size adult mannequin that allowed students to practice fundamental nursing skills. Mrs. Martha Chase designed Mrs. Chase for the Hartford Hospital Nurse Training program in Hartford, Connecticut, and it became part of nursing education in 1911 (Singleton 2020). She was considered quite sophisticated with her realistic movable joints and parts. She was a model patient who endured baths, bandaging, dressing changes, turning, bedmaking, warm and cold compresses, and positioning.

We also learned by practicing on our fellow students. By bathing each other, we learned to bathe our patients. In addition to teaching us the actual skill, we learned firsthand what the patients experienced and how they might feel, resulting in a more compassionate approach. By administering injections to each other, we learned how to inject patients. Starting intravenous access (IVs) on each other taught us how to start them on patients. This promoted empathy for the patient's feelings as they received care, and we learned the importance of kindness and a gentle touch. My "little sis" went above and beyond when she volunteered to receive an enema in front of her class for the enema day learning experience.

After much anxious anticipation, the day of our first clinical finally arrived. Our class filled the tunnel with nervous, animated chatter as we proceeded to our assigned ward dressed in our neatly pressed student uniforms. Student uniforms consisted of a one-piece white pinafore over a light blue blouse. The material was a comfortable cotton/polyester. We would not have dared report to clinicals in a wrinkled uniform. The only jewelry allowed was a watch with a working second hand to calculate pulse, respirations, and IV drips. Our red and black ink pens and bandage scissors were secured in a small plastic carrying case to prevent ink from "bleeding" through our uniform pocket. Married students were allowed to wear a plain wedding ring. Otherwise, jewelry was not allowed. If you think anyone might have had a tattoo, think again. Because our hair could not touch the collar of our uniforms, those with long hair learned how to style it attractively pinned up off the collar.

Spending most of our time on our feet, we quickly learned the importance of supportive shoes and hose. Good white support hose and white nursing oxfords were paramount to working long hours standing and walking. Because of the strong vertical elasticity, they were prone to "ride down" as they compressed and facilitated circulation.

We hoped our hose remained at our waist because migrating support hose sliding over our hips was uncomfortable and made working difficult. The recommended way to put them on was to gather one leg of the hose in your hand. The toe would be inserted into the stocking portion, and the hose would be eased up your leg with gentle pulling. Pulling too hard risked creating a run or a hole in the stocking. Should that happen, that pair was ruined and had to be replaced. Ideally, the leg was elevated during this donning process to aid circulation and venous return up the leg. Extra points were awarded if you could lie on your back and do this. The goal was to obtain support from the ankle to the top of the thigh to promote good circulation and minimize leg fatigue. White "nurse" support hosiery was easily acquired then. I found that only Nurse Mates currently manufactures this hosiery.

Everyone wore white Oxford lace-up shoes, usually Clinic or Stride Rite brands. Clinic shoes offered the most support and were the chosen brand for most of us. They were not cheap, and given the amount of time spent on our feet, a new pair was required annually. Nike, Skechers, or other "sneakers" did not exist and wouldn't have been allowed. Clean, polished shoes free of dirt and scuff marks were required. After applying white shoe polish, we buffed them to retain the shine. Our name tag and nursing cap indicating our level of education finished off our uniform. Our name tags included our first and last names, but we were to introduce ourselves using only our surnames, such as Miss or Mrs., and our last name. No Ms. at that time.

Because my maiden name was Ethell, it was not uncommon for me to introduce myself as Miss Ethell and be asked, "What's your last name"? Ethell. First-year students wore a plain white nurse's cap, second-year students had a narrow vertical black stripe on one side of the cap, third-year students sported a black stripe across the cap, and remained our permanent nursing cap after graduation. Caps were secured to our hair by white bobby pins, two on each side at the back of the cap and one in the front middle to prevent them from flopping around or falling off. I proudly wore my cap without attaching any negativity to it. By the 1980's the nursing cap was rarely worn. I still hear physicians and patients state they wish nurses wore caps because it was an easy, straightforward way to identify the nurses on the unit.

In her book, Celebrating Nurses: A Visual History, Dr. Christine Hallett states, "Nurses' caps reflect the changing story of nursing by showing how nurses were perceived, and what their role in society was at different times" (Hallett, 2010, p. 96). She says nurses' caps evolved from the nuns' coif and were made from starched, white material. As we learned more about germs, the cap was seen as a way of keeping hair out of the eyes and preventing contamination of sterile fields. Caps were unique to one's school of nursing so one could distinguish the school the nurse graduated from by looking at her nurse's cap.

Throughout my education, nurses wore white uniforms – dresses or two-piece pantsuits. Scrub attire was only worn in the Operating Room (OR), and those scrubs were dresses. White uniforms were available in many department stores and "uniform" stores offering numerous attractive styles. White nursing shoes and hose were usually available in those stores. I recall purchasing my nursing shoes at shoe stores and hose at a local department store. I believe they could also be purchased through JCPenney or Sears catalogs.

I do not recall nurses having much autonomy during my nursing education. Doctors gave orders, and nurses followed them. Questioning a doctor's order did not occur without a compelling reason to do so. I doubt that recommendations from a nurse regarding patient care would have been readily sought or accepted. Although physicians were usually congenial towards the nursing staff, the concept of a robust, productive, collaborative nurse-physician team was yet to come.

Because doctors can and do make mistakes, our class discussed when it might be appropriate to question a physician's order. For example, a nurse might question a medication order beyond the normal dose or other instances of "off-ness". We shared a situation where a patient experienced a cardiac arrest, and the physician defibrillated the patient several times (nurses were not allowed to independently defibrillate patients as they are today). For example, we will assume that the standard of care at that time was to defibrillate twice. When the life-saving measures resulted in the patient surviving, the STUDENT NURSE questioned the doctor. She reportedly said the literature supports defibrillating twice, but he had defibrillated three times (also not today's practice). Because this doctor was known to be gruff with an intimidating, booming voice that resonated on the unit, we were aghast that she would question him. We were especially stunned at her assertiveness towards THIS physician after he had just saved the patient's life. Thankfully, he found her "brazenness" humorous and laughed about the incident. Fortunately, she lived to graduate.

Unlike today's short (or no) hospital stays, patients remained hospitalized for as long as the doctor deemed necessary. Ten-day hospital stays were not unusual, especially following major surgery. Even patients having minor surgery might be hospitalized for three to five days.

Procedures considered outpatient today required an inpatient stay of several days. For instance, patients were often on bed rest for a day or two after eye surgery, then allowed to dangle on the side of the bed, progress to sitting in a chair, and finally walk in the hallway before discharge. Other surgical procedures allowed patients to remain in bed longer than is currently practiced. Suffice it to say we weren't as aggressive in ambulating post-operative patients as we are today. This lack of postoperative activity predisposed patients to dangerous side effects such as pneumonia, constipation, and blood clots that were life-threatening if they traveled to the lungs (pulmonary embolism).

Patients with fractures, such as broken arms or legs, did not have the sophisticated pins and plate instrumentation available today. Although instrumentation to fix a fractured hip was available and used, patients often spent sustained periods in traction as hospital inpatients waiting for their fractures to heal. I recall having a hospitalized patient imprisoned in a full-body cast for months. It is hard to imagine being immobilized for that length of time, dressed only in a hospital gown, dependent on others for everything, without control of any aspect of your life.

Patients scheduled for major or minor surgery were hospitalized the night before their procedure. The surgical site and surrounding area were shaved with a razor the night before the surgery. Today, the surgical incision is minimally cleared of hair using a clipper. Shaving the night before and using a razor increases the chance of a post-operative infection. Razors cause small nicks in the skin, increasing the risk of introducing bacteria into the surgical wound when the incision is made. Other preoperative preparations might require administering enemas until clear the night before.

Patients undergoing multiple tests could be admitted to the hospital until the tests were completed. Before diagnostic-related groups dictated reimbursement for diagnoses or procedures, hospitals could bill insurance for the hospital stay with little accountability for the length of that stay.

With that in mind, living adjacent to the hospital, we students had the advantage of direct access to our patients' information the night before our clinical experience. Because we received our patient assignments the night before our clinical, the patients' presence on the unit provided ample time to study their medical records. We were required to prepare for the next day's clinical by reviewing the patient's chart, including history and physical, progress notes, test results, implications for scheduled procedures and tests, treatment plan, medications, and the Kardex. Nursing textbooks and other resources were used to assimilate the information we had gathered into a nursing care plan encompassing physical, psychological, social, and cultural elements.

The care we provided reflected our educational and skill level at that time. During those early days, our instructor constantly guided us through each step, ensuring its proper completion. As new students, we worked more slowly and deliberately than the employed nursing staff, making sure each step was correctly completed.

Nursing is often compartmentalized into skills such as bathing patients, cleaning bedpans, giving oral medications and injections, starting IVs, using hot or cold compresses, or administering enemas. While those skills are part of hands-on nursing care, nursing encompasses much more than that. Nurses develop keen observation skills which can literally save the patient's life. They assess the body's response to illness by anticipating and identifying physiological and psychological responses connected to the patient's diagnosis. Nurses are adept at identifying symptoms the patient is exhibiting, formulating a nursing diagnosis, communicating those observations to the physician, anticipating the intervention, and administering the appropriate treatment prescribed.

The American Nurses Association describes nursing as a "health care profession that integrates the art and science of caring and focuses on the protection, promotion, and optimization of health and human functioning; prevention of illness and injury; facilitation of healing; and alleviation of suffering through compassionate presence" (Association, American Nurses, 2021, p. 1). Physicians focus on diagnosis and treating the disease process, but nurses focus on caring for the patient. To provide that care, nurses possess vast knowledge about the human body, disease processes, pharmacology, and medical and surgical treatment modalities.

Nurses understand how various medications work in the body and observe the body's response to those medications, knowing what to look for and how the patient is expected to respond. This knowledge allows them to separate normal vs abnormal responses. Nurses are knowledgeable regarding the myriad of surgical interventions, the expected effects of that surgery, and normal and abnormal responses to the surgery. Nurses possess an anticipatory awareness of what to look for in patients undergoing surgery. A nurse's knowledge allows them to anticipate and prepare for the next steps in the patient's treatment plan.

As students, we learned how to incorporate the patient's information to create an individual nursing care plan for each patient. Our care plans reflected our level of knowledge and skill. As we progressed through nursing education, the care plans became increasingly complex and detailed.

Nursing care plans were created using the Nursing Process of Assessment, Diagnosis, Planning, Implementation, and Evaluation. The assessment includes gathering relevant data and pertinent information by reviewing the patient's medical record, including prescribed medications, examining and interviewing the patient to obtain a history, and observing clinical signs. Once gathered, the information is assimilated to form a picture of the patient's condition. We identified pertinent aspects of the patient's condition and "diagnosed" the nursing care we anticipated would be required to care for that patient. We then planned the nursing care related to the diagnosis and our findings. We defended our nursing diagnosis by documenting the "Scientific Principles Underlying Patient Care" in the care plan beside each diagnosis. In other words, what evidence was used to formulate our nursing diagnosis? How did we know that our plan was the correct course of action? The scientific principles supported the plan, which included goals and outcomes that the patient would attain based on the diagnosis and nursing care. The plan was implemented as part of our care for the patient. For instance, for a patient undergoing surgery, one diagnosis would consider that the anesthetic impacts the patient's respiratory tract, which contributes to the development of postoperative pneumonia. With that knowledge, how would we as nurses prevent it? We PLANNED to assist the patient in taking deep breaths and coughing at regular intervals to clear the lungs. Upon the patient's return to the unit after surgery, the above plan was implemented. The evaluation determined the results of the above steps and answered the question as to whether we had correctly assessed the patient, planned the appropriate care, and effectively implemented that care. The evaluation validated whether we had achieved the desired outcome by monitoring the patient's response to our nursing care. If the surgical patient recovered from the surgery without complications from pneumonia, we had achieved that goal. If the patient were bedridden, the nursing care plan would identify the need to prevent pressure ulcers by turning the patient at regular intervals, keeping the patient clean and dry, bathing the patient and applying lotion, avoiding friction injury, etc. The evaluation would tell us if those interventions had been successful. Did the patient indeed avoid bed sores and pressure ulcers?

Our handwritten nursing care plan was turned in to our instructor the following day. She reviewed the care plan, made appropriate notations, and graded it. The complexity of the care plan reflected our level of education, clinical skill, and expected nursing judgment. By senior year, our care plans might be several pages in length.

I have used the principles of the nursing care plan throughout my career. When I was doing bedside and surgical nursing, I applied it to individual patients. When I moved into an administrative role, I used it to assess and build my team, or create change. It was an invaluable tool throughout my career, and relevant at many levels. Situations changed, but the principles and processes remained the same.

Compared to the current technology available to the medical community, 1970s technology was ancient. An electric typewriter was a luxury. Most documentation was accomplished by pen, pencils, and paper – nurse's notes, progress notes, physician orders, and the Kardex. In her article, *A Look at Hospital Nursing During the 1970s*, Frieda Paton states, "You would feel lost and confused if you were transported back in time to a hospital ward in the 1970s when the nurses who are now at the end of their careers were students". She points out that the "world has changed dramatically over the past few decades, and most of the changes are the result of the growth in knowledge and technology. Towards the beginning of the 1900s, knowledge was doubling about every 100 years; after World War II, it was doubling every 25 years, and it is estimated that knowledge currently doubles on average every 13 months" (Paton, 2021, p. 1). It is no wonder that today's nursing profession barely resembles what it was like when I entered it in 1968.

The lack of computers meant documenting everything manually. The patient's medical record was organized in an aluminum patient chart clipboard housed in a rotating chart holder, which was centrally located at the nurse's station. Allergies were noted with a piece of red and white tape affixed to the front of the chart. The front of the chart might contain other taped reminders, such as NPO (food and water held). The charts were readily available to the entire medical team and arranged in chronological order according to patient room number. The unit secretary who was assigned to each patient care area kept the charts in order. Patients with extensive hospitalizations might have a thick chart that the Unit Secretary would periodically "thin". When the physician arrived on the unit, the secretary had all of the doctor's charts available for him/her to review and write orders. Requisitions were completed on typewriters, and the hard copy was sent by pneumatic tube to the appropriate department or hand-carried to that department when the Unit Secretary ran errands.

The Kardex was the precursor to today's electronic medical record. In her article in American Nurse Today, Pamela F. Cipriano states, "Nurses lived and died by the Kardex, a folded card-stock roadmap to all things for the patient. It was completed in pencil and continuously crossed out or erased and updated" (Cipriano, 2010, p. 1). Each card resided in a flip folder containing every patient in the nursing unit. Cards were arranged according to room number and provided a snapshot of the patient and his/her hospital stay. Patient information included the patient's name, age, marital status, religious preference, allergies, chief complaints, reason for admission, medical diagnosis, resuscitation code, list of medications, treatments, diet, IV therapy/medications, activity status, and upcoming tests or procedures. It allowed nurses a readily accessible reference for each patient. The Kardex was updated as needed to reflect the current patient status or changes.

Nursing shifts were eight hours. To my knowledge, ten and twelve-hour shifts did not exist, at least not at Mennonite. The day shift was 7 AM to 3:30 PM, the evening shift was 3 PM to 11:30 PM, and the night shift was 11:00 PM to 7:30 AM. The half-hour overlap accommodated the report for each shift. The oncoming shift assembled in the conference room for the change-of-shift report. The outgoing charge RN reported on each patient by flipping to the Kardex page for that patient. A hypothetical report would go something like this: "This is Mr. John Smith, room 305, bed 1, a 50-year-old patient of Dr. Johnson, admitted to the hospital on June 15 with abdominal pain. He is allergic to penicillin, etc. ". She would then review the patient status for that particular day and shift. Tests that were completed that day, test results if available, medications he's on and the response to those medications, IV fluid and the rate, how he tolerated his diet, ambulation, any communication with the doctor, vital signs, and information the oncoming shift might need to check. The Kardex contributed to the successful achievement of continuity of care. New doctor's orders were signed off by the RN and entered into the Kardex for the care team to review. Entries were made in pencil because it was a fluid document to be revised as needed. The Kardex was not part of the patient's medical record (Ang, 2019 Mount-Campbell et al., 2020).

Team nursing served as the model for patient care, with teams led by an RN team leader. Each team was responsible for a specific number of patients, often encompassing as many as half the ward. RNs handled patient care that required a professional nursing license. Their duties included coordinating and overseeing the care provided by their team, administering medications, managing IV fluids, delivering treatments, rounding with physicians, and conducting team meetings for certain patients. Nursing Assistants and LPNs took care of the remaining duties, such as bathing, making beds, assisting patients into chairs, and taking vital signs as dictated by patient acuity.

As students, we attended the change of shift report and received information about our patients. We arrived on the unit with the employed nursing staff and listened as the Charge RN reported on each patient housed on that unit. We might work in tandem with the hospital staff, but we essentially provided patient care according to our educational and skill level.

As previously stated, everything was written by hand. We "charted" the care we provided by documenting everything pertinent to that patient in the nurse's notes on the patient's chart. Because the written entries were narrative, nursing documentation on a higher acuity patient was long and descriptive as we diligently included every detail of the patient care we provided. There were no boxes to simply check off the nursing interventions. We understood the importance of creating a picture of the care the patient received and the patient's response to that care.

The chart is a legal document, meaning that anything written in it is admissible in court or other legal proceedings. Only medically recognized abbreviations were to be used. Everything documented had a prescribed way of doing it. All chart entries began with the date and time care was administered. When the charting entry was complete, we signed our names and professional status. My chart entry was signed Ila Ethell, SN for student nurse. Our handwriting was checked to make sure it was legible. Before leaving the unit, we reported to the oncoming nurse and completed the patient "handoff". As we neared graduation towards the end of our senior year, we learned the team leader role and reported for that entire team to the oncoming shift.

Our nursing instructor was present in the unit and oversaw everything we did to ensure consistency in our clinical education. Morning care included taking vital signs, preparing the patient for breakfast, feeding the patient if necessary, giving a complete bath (our patients were bathed with soap and water unlike today's bath in a bag), administering medications, completing treatments, preparing the patient for surgery if required, and monitoring the patient post-operatively or post-procedure.

Preparing the patient for breakfast included offering a damp washcloth to wipe their face and hands, and assisting them with brushing their teeth. The food service department was not responsible for delivering the tray to the patient's room or setting it up. They delivered the cart containing the trays of food to the unit, and the nursing staff passed them out. Based on information from the morning report, nursing staff were assigned to patients requiring feeding before the shift began. Because of our hospital's affiliation with Gailey Eye Clinic, we performed a lot of eye surgery, so it was not unusual for patients to have one or both eyes bandaged. We learned to feed blindfolded patients unable to feed themselves by being blindfolded and having our partner feed us. We would then switch so we all experienced what it was like to be the person feeding and the person being fed.

Before the arrival of the breakfast tray, if the patient was self-fed, we raised the head of the bed or assisted the patient to a chair to eat. We never placed the tray on the bedside table and left the room, leaving the patients to fend for themselves. When we brought the tray, we "set it up" meaning we removed all the lids, opened the milk carton, prepared the cereal and coffee according to the patient's instructions, salted and peppered as directed, took silverware out of the protective cover, opened straws and placed in the drinks, and cut food as patient condition required. We prepared everything. If the patient required feeding, the student remained in the room and fed the patient. This often required a great deal of time. As students, we had time to do this correctly. However, as a nurse on a busy unit with limited staff, feeding patients could be a challenging undertaking. When each meal was completed, the nursing staff collected the trays and documented how well the patient ate. If the patient's intake was being monitored, we documented the amounts of each liquid consumed.

  Following breakfast, we bathed our patient(s). The patient's bath was quite involved because we were taught the importance of the bath for healing and observation. Supplies for a bed bath included a round metal basin, soap, a towel, and a washcloth. The water was tested for proper temperature, making sure it wasn't too hot. The patient was disrobed and covered with a flannel bath sheet. The washcloth was folded around our hand to form a mitt, which prevented the edges of the washcloth from flopping around. The bed bath started with the face and neck. We then placed an unfolded towel under the patient's arm. We washed and rinsed the arm, wrapped the towel around it, and patted it dry. The skin was not rubbed with the towel because that would promote skin breakdown. The process was repeated with the other arm. We covered the chest and abdomen with a towel before lowering the bath sheet. To maintain the female patient's privacy, we carefully lifted the towel to wash the chest and abdomen and replaced the towel with each step. Therefore, the patient was minimally exposed during this portion of the bath. A towel was placed beneath each leg as it was washed and rinsed. Each leg was dried similarly, with the towel wrapped around the leg to pat it dry. A towel was placed under each foot, and the patient's foot was placed in the basin of water to wash it. After both feet were washed, the water was changed. The patient was then rolled to one side, either on their own or someone held them over and supported them so the back could be washed. To prevent skin breakdown, after washing and drying, we rubbed lotion over the entire back to stimulate circulation and promote comfort. It was then time to "finish the bath," which meant washing the genitalia. The patient was asked if they could "finish" their own bath. If yes, we would hold a towel up to provide privacy and hand them the washcloth with soap, rinse it, and hand the washcloth back to them, then dry. If they were unable to "finish" their own bath, we did it. However, females only touched female patients. We summoned a male orderly to assist the men. If the patient was well enough to sit in the chair, they were assisted out of bed, making it easier for us to make the bed. Otherwise, we made the bed with the patient in it. There were no fitted sheets, so the bottom sheet and the draw sheet were tucked in tightly to prevent them from coming loose from the bed. The pillowcase was changed by turning it inside out, grasping the end of the pillow while holding onto the pillowcase, and sliding the pillowcase over the pillow. We were taught the importance of not stirring up dust in the room, so pillows were never shaken down into the pillowcase. When the pillow was returned to the bed, it was placed with the open end facing away from the door to provide a neater appearance for anyone entering the room. Bed linen was changed daily – all of it. When the bath was finished, we positioned the patient, ensured they were comfortable, straightened their bedside area, provided fresh water, and placed the call light within the patient's immediate reach.

Vital signs or TPR (temperature, pulse, respiration) and blood pressure were taken manually. Each patient's mercury thermometer was housed in an individual holder. As student nurses, we quickly learned the difference between rectal and oral thermometers. Oral thermometers were plain, and rectal thermometers had a red area at the end of the thermometer. Before taking the patient's temperature, the thermometer was "shaken down" by holding the thermometer and snapping our wrists to shake down the mercury. After verifying that the patient had not recently ingested anything hot or cold that would affect the temperature, the thermometer was placed under the patient's tongue. Axillary or rectal temperatures were obtained for patients who risked biting down on the thermometer or were too ill to hold it under their tongue. A degree was added to axillary temperatures and subtracted from the rectal temperatures obtained.

Using the second hand on our watch, we learned to palpate a radial pulse and count the beats. If it was a routine check, the beats were counted for 15 seconds and multiplied by four. However, if the patient had been prescribed heart medication, the beats were counted for an entire minute. Patients with a heart issue might require checking an apical-radial pulse, which requires palpating the radial artery while placing the stethoscope over the heart and counting the beats to ensure the radial pulse matches the heartbeat. When calculating respirations, we continued holding our fingers over the radial pulse to make it appear like we were counting the heart rate. Although to the patient it looked like we were palpating the pulse, we were actually observing the chest rising and counting the respirations. The respiratory rate might be incorrect if the patient was aware of being watched while breathing. These results were transcribed in graph form by the Unit Secretary on the patient's chart.

Blood pressure was calculated manually using a sphygmomanometer and a stethoscope. Digital, automated blood pressure monitors did not exist. Practicing on one another helped us get accustomed to the rising and fading of the lub-dub sound. The first beat indicated the systolic or upper number, and the last beat heard was the diastolic or lower number. Identifying extraneous sounds and other abnormalities took time to perfect. Learning these skills took time because the actions of the students were deliberate, as the instructor closely observed us diligently striving for a correct outcome.

Speaking of enemas, the enemas administered contained water with a packet of castile soap. There was a receptacle for water and a long plastic tube with several "tick" marks on it. After filling the receptacle with approximately a quart of warm water, the soap was added. The "tick" marks measured how far the plastic tube was inserted into the rectum. The receptacle hung on an IV pole while the water was slowly infused. If the patient experienced discomfort, the tubing was clamped until the discomfort subsided before proceeding with the enema. The castile soap acted as a bowel irritant to stimulate evacuation. This procedure was exhausting for weak or debilitated patients. Although students would not have administered them, some enemas were ordered as 3-H – High, Hot, and Heck of a lot for patients with stubborn constipation issues.

Due to the time required for ISU classes, first-year clinical time was limited to three hours one morning per week. Having received patient assignments the afternoon before, we went to the unit to review the patient's chart and develop a care plan. Three hours allowed enough time to conduct morning vitals, bathe the patient, and assist with feeding if needed.

Because passing medications involved more than administering pills and giving shots, we were also enrolled in a Pharmacology class. Wikipedia defines Pharmacology as 'the science of drugs and medications, including a substance's origin, composition, pharmacokinetics, pharmacodynamics, therapeutic use, and toxicology. More specifically, it studies the interactions between a living organism and chemicals that affect normal or abnormal biochemical function. Substances with medicinal properties are considered pharmaceuticals" (Pharmacology, 2024, p. 1). The pharmacology class taught the theory and technique for administering medications.

The different "classes" of medication were studied, including blood pressure, cardiovascular, antibiotics, pain medications, steroids, anticoagulants, vasoconstrictors (medications that constrict the blood vessels), vasodilators (medications that dilate the blood vessels), etc. We then learned about specific medications in each class and their impact on the human body. We were expected to articulate the correct mode of administration, time required for the medication's peak action, half-life, how the medication was metabolized, side effects, adverse reactions, and contraindications. If the nurse gave an IV medication, how should it be administered – drip or IV push? If it came in a powder form, how was it reconstituted – water or saline, and the amount used? As students, we were quizzed and tested on all of this information. How did the medication affect the bodily organs such as the liver, kidneys, or circulatory system? How was the medication metabolized? We learned the effects of the class of medications and the action of specific medications. What were their contraindications – when shouldn't they be given? We learned how to anticipate, recognize, and treat adverse reactions.

Back then, nurses often calculated doses themselves. If a medication came in one dose, but a lower dose was ordered, the nurse was taught how to calculate the ordered dose. Today, those calculations are the responsibility of the pharmacist. The pharmacy did not coordinate or oversee the mixing of medications. They dispensed medication to the unit without coordinating medication administration, as is the case today. Nurses mixed their IV medications, including antibiotics, without assistance from the Pharmacist.

Each unit had a Physician's Desk Reference (PDR) and the U.S. Pharmacopeia, huge hard-cover books containing every available medication. The PDR was an annual publication listing each medication's generic and trade names with detailed descriptions of every drug. These thick, cumbersome books were the main source of information about the patients' medications. To make these references readily available for everyone, the books were frequently chained to the desk at the nurse's station to avoid them "walking off".

We memorized an extensive list of Pharmacological abbreviations, many of which are no longer used today due to the risk of misreading the abbreviation, leading to serious medical error. Poor penmanship was a major factor in misreading a medication dose. For instance, q.d. means every day, and q.i.d. means four times a day – easily misread. OS, OD, and OU mean left eye, right eye, or both eyes. MS and MS04 – one means morphine sulfate, while the other means magnesium sulfate, two different substances. One can see how easily it would be to misread the order. Each order was meticulously reviewed. Today's regulations dictate that almost all orders are written and transcribed longhand.

Medications might be dispensed via a medication cart that was rolled from room to room by the RN in charge of those patients. Each patient had a drawer of medications. Any adjustment of medication dose was completed by the nurse. Each patient's medication order was listed on a typed Medication Administration Record (MAR) contained in the medication Kardex housed on the medication cart. However, I recall filling medications in the "medication room" and placing patients' medications on a tray. Oral medications would be placed in a cup contained in a little holder with the patient's name. Injections were labeled and also placed on the tray. Talk about a recipe for disaster!

  As students, before we could administer medication, we researched the specific medication, identified its physiological purpose, the proper mode of administration, how it was to be administered, i.e. with meals, etc., and all side effects. This information was written on index cards, which were filed in our little recipe box under headings such as "pain medication", blood pressure", and "anti-coagulants". This provided us with a library of sorts for each medication administered. As our "library" grew, we used the index cards as a reference. The patient's medications were documented on the patient's care plan that we prepared, including mode of action, appropriate dose, side effects, and adverse reactions. We were quizzed on all of these points before the medication was administered to the patient.

  Because we were novice first-year students, medication administration was a very tedious process. We verified the patient's identification by comparing the patient's identification band with the medication administration record. This ensured the dose aligned with the physician's order, ensuring the correct route of administration, identifying any patient allergies, and ensuring it was administered at the time and interval ordered. The nurse was responsible for monitoring the drug's effect on the patient. The nurses' notes reflected the patient's tolerance of the drug and any side effects they exhibited. The patient was monitored for signs that the drug had achieved its therapeutic purpose. For example, if the patient received a medication to lower his/her blood pressure (B/P), the patient's B/P was taken before administering the medication. Following the prescribed amount of time for the drug to work, the patient's blood pressure was retaken to determine if the drug had the desired effect on the patient's B/P.

Before dismissal for spring break freshman year, we learned to administer intramuscular (IM) injections by giving IM injections of saline to each other. Most people dislike receiving injections, so the thought of receiving one from someone who had never given one was somewhat unsettling. We also feared giving an injection to our friends. Hopefully, they would remain our friends following this exercise. Because the syringes contained saline, the injections were not painful. We learned the correct technique for filling the syringe with the medication, identifying the appropriate anatomical location, and the best technique for causing the least amount of discomfort when the needle punctured the skin. By the end of freshman year, we were administering oral medications and intramuscular injections.

Sophisticated medical equipment was not as prevalent as it is today. Regular patient rooms did not have built-in oxygen or suction. Those luxuries were reserved for patients residing in the Intensive Care Unit (ICU). Regular rooms required an oxygen tank to be rolled into the room for patients requiring oxygen. Tanks were monitored and changed when the oxygen ran low.

Patient rooms in the older section of the hospital lacked modern conveniences such as a toilet. Each room had a sink. Although the newly constructed wing boasted toilets in each patient room, they were absent from the older section of the hospital. Patients used bedpans or bedside commodes if they were allowed. With no toilet, bedpan or commode contents were covered with a towel and taken to the dirty utility room, where they were emptied into the hopper. And remember, we did not wear gloves. Ambulatory patients could walk down the hall to the patient bathroom located there.

There were very few private patient rooms. Most patient rooms were double occupancy. Some patient units contained multi-bed wards with up to four patient beds. Not only did hospitalized patients not feel well, but they also lost all semblance of privacy.

Suction was accomplished using an electric Gomco suction machine obtained from Central Supply and assigned to the patient. The regulator valve provided the correct amount of suction. The drainage from the patient was collected in a reusable glass jar. At the end of each shift, the glass jar was disconnected from the machine, the contents were measured, and the glass jar was covered with a towel to conceal it as it was carried to the dirty utility room to be discarded in the hopper. The nurse charted the amount and description of the drainage in the nurse's notes. When suction was no longer required, the unit was returned to Central Service to be cleaned and readied for the next patient.

There were no computers, no Pyxus, no digital thermometers, and no electronic blood pressure machines. Patients' cardiac status was not monitored unless they were patients in the Intensive Care Unit (ICU). Cardiac monitors were frequently portable. Everything was done manually, including operating some of the beds. Manual beds in the older wing contained three cranks at the foot of the bed to be operated by hand. One crank raised the head of the bed, one raised the foot, and one raised and lowered the entire bed. These beds required the nursing staff to engage in substantial manual labor. The patient had no control over their position, so if they wanted their head or foot raised or lowered, they activated their call light and waited for someone to come and help them. Again, the newly constructed wing did have electric hospital beds capable of being operated by the patient.

Because we did not complete a head-to-toe assessment on the patient, I did not hone those skills until 1981 when I worked in the Coronary Care Unit (CCU). Although we learned the individual components of the nursing assessment such as taking apical/radial pulses, auscultating the heart, stages of edema, neurological signs, etc., the actual head-to-toe assessment of listening and identifying heart sounds, lung sounds, bowel sounds, and conducting a complete head-to-toe assessment on admission or at the change of shift were not completed at that time.

Before the arrival of HIV/AIDS around 1981, we did not wear gloves when handling bedpans, emesis basins, diapers, soiled dressings, colostomy bags, bloody dressings, urine from a Foley catheter bag, or anything else containing body fluids. I remain traumatized recalling cleaning vomited chili out of a patient's bathroom sink. We just took a deep breath and got it done. We did not want the patient to feel embarrassed that their bodily functions were repulsive or difficult for us, although they were, in fact, repulsive and difficult for us. Nor did we wear protective eyewear for anything, including the operating room. If you got splashed or squirted in the eye, you got splashed or squirted in the eye. Wipe it out and continue working. We were expected to perform our jobs and tend to the patient's needs, whatever that required. To be a nurse and work in healthcare, one had to make peace with soiled hands that required frequent washing.

Universal precautions did not exist. The infection control protocol was based on the organism cultured. Although it was best practice for healthcare workers to wash their hands after each patient, this practice certainly was not strictly followed. Healthcare workers sometimes moved from room to room caring for patient after patient without adherence to strict handwashing. Hand sanitizer did not exist. Hands were sanitized by washing with soap and water.

In the spring of my freshman year, I was hired part-time to work at the hospital switchboard, a wonderful opportunity I enjoyed until graduation. I worked every other weekend. Saturday was a split shift requiring me to work 8 AM to 12:30 PM, leave for the afternoon, and return 5 PM to 9 PM. On Sundays I worked from 12 PM to 8:30 PM. Those shifts worked fine during the school year, but in August, when school was not in session, I drove the 60 minutes home on dark country roads with no means to communicate with my parents if I experienced difficulty. Because I did not own a car until I got married, I drove my parents' only vehicle to and from work.

Forget about today's modern technology. We wore a headset while working with a switchboard in front of us. As calls came into the hospital, we "connected" them to the appropriate extension. The "paging" system featured a microphone that was activated by pushing a lever, allowing the switchboard operator to speak into the microphone to transmit our voice throughout the hospital. We often doubled as the information desk for guests entering the hospital. Working "off hours" provided some interesting experiences. Being a moderate-sized community hospital, we did not have a large Emergency Room (ER). It consisted of one major room and a few rooms designated for minor things. Immediate or Urgent Care facilities outside of the doctor's office did not exist then, so everything came through the Emergency Room. If a high-acuity patient was brought in, he/she was transferred to a larger facility. Our Emergency Room wasn't staffed evenings or weekends.

The switchboard window looked out onto the hospital's emergency entrance, which the ambulances accessed via the physician parking lot. During those unstaffed hours, when we saw an ambulance entering the parking lot, we overhead-paged the Nursing Supervisor to the Emergency Room to begin care. Because we received no notification that the ambulance was coming, it was our job to keep a sharp lookout in anticipation of its potential arrival. Sometimes, we would get busy and spontaneously look out the window, "Oh! There's an ambulance!"

The ER was located a short distance from the switchboard, literally down the hall and around the corner. Therefore, if the Nursing Supervisor was busy and not readily available, the switchboard operator went to the ER to at least welcome the patient. Can you imagine being ill enough to come to the ER and asking the first person you see if they are a nurse or a doctor? "No, I'm the switchboard operator". One of the operators LOVED being the first responder to the ER. If the Nursing Supervisor didn't come right away, she would make a beeline to the ER to find out what was going on. Once the Nursing Supervisor arrived, she would return to the switchboard and report what was happening.

Weekends at the switchboard could be rather slow, resulting in boredom. And I'm ashamed to say that if it was a slow Saturday night, we may or may not have participated in prank calls to the local fraternities and Lucas Bar and Grill.

I loved working the switchboard with wonderful coworkers who became friends throughout my time at Mennonite. One of my coworkers manned the switchboard for over 50 years and was recognized in the local newspaper around 2014 when she was 92 years old and still working.

**Summer School ISU 1969**

Most of our college credits were obtained during the first and second semesters of our freshman year with two remaining classes for the first semester of our junior year. I elected to attend summer school at ISU to obtain those junior-year credits. I wanted to experience college life, and I thought it would give me a "jump start" to my junior year of nursing school. An added perk meant I avoided riding Virgil. One of my fellow nursing students made the same decision, allowing us to room together at Hewitt Hall on the ISU campus. I enjoyed the summer living in the large dorm, meeting people, and making new friends.

Little did I know how that decision would impact the rest of my life because I met my future husband during summer school. My friend in the room next to mine received an impromptu call from one of her friends asking her if she was available for a blind date. She declined and came to our room, asking if one of us would like to go. I agreed to go and promptly went to the dorm lobby, where I was met by two other couples (one being my future husband and his date) and my date, who greeted me sporting bilateral leg casts for not one but two broken legs sustained during a skydiving mishap. It was a decent evening, and I had a nice time. The following day, I received a call from Terry (my future husband), inviting me to go out with him. Our first date occurred on July 20, 1969, when Apollo Eleven landed on the moon, making it easy to remember throughout our married life. Although I wasn't looking for a Christian boyfriend, the guy I met in summer school, who later became my husband, was also a Christian. We have been together for over 50 years.

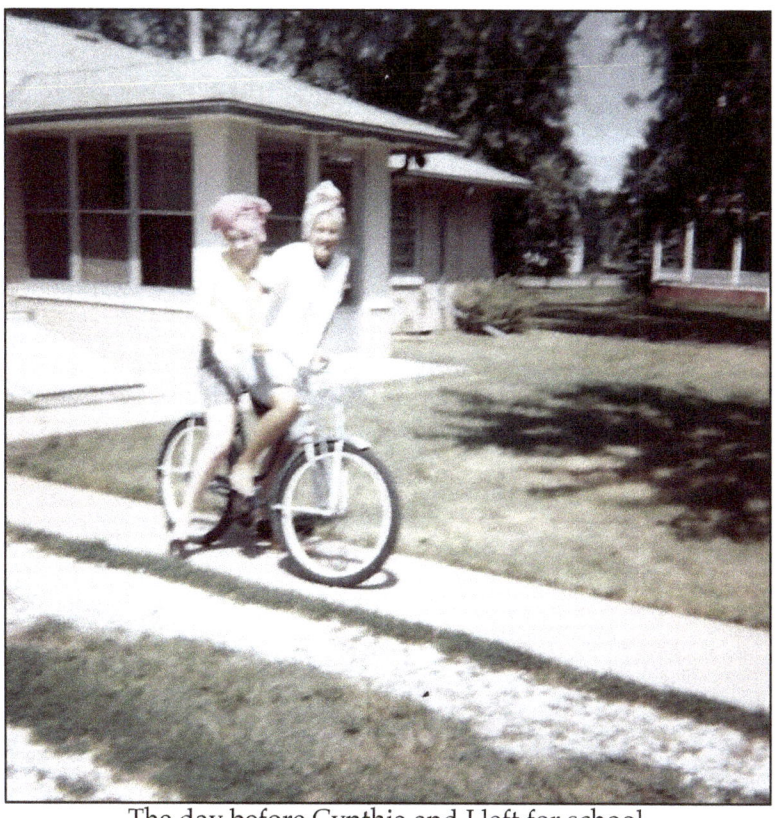
The day before Cynthia and I left for school

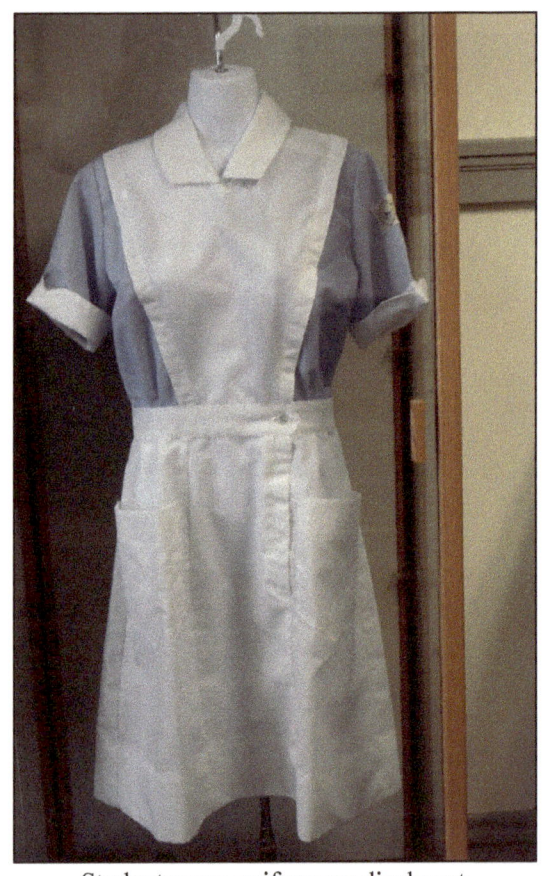

Student nurse uniform on display at
Mennonite College of Nursing,
Illinois State University

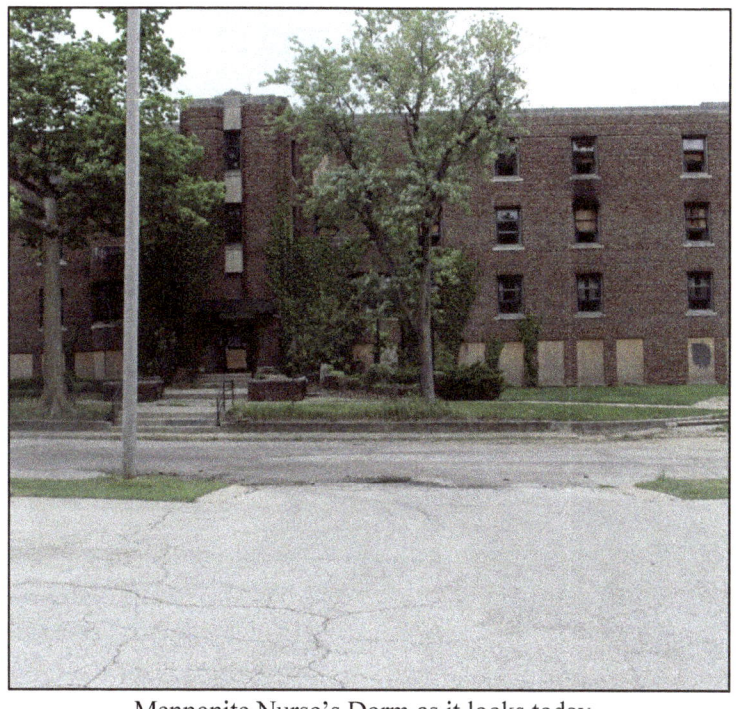

Mennonite Nurse's Dorm as it looks today.
My "big sis" was waiting for me on the first landing
when I arrived at Mennonite with my parents.

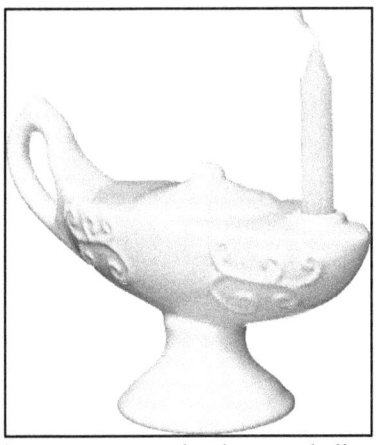

The Nightingale Lamp we received at our dedication ceremony

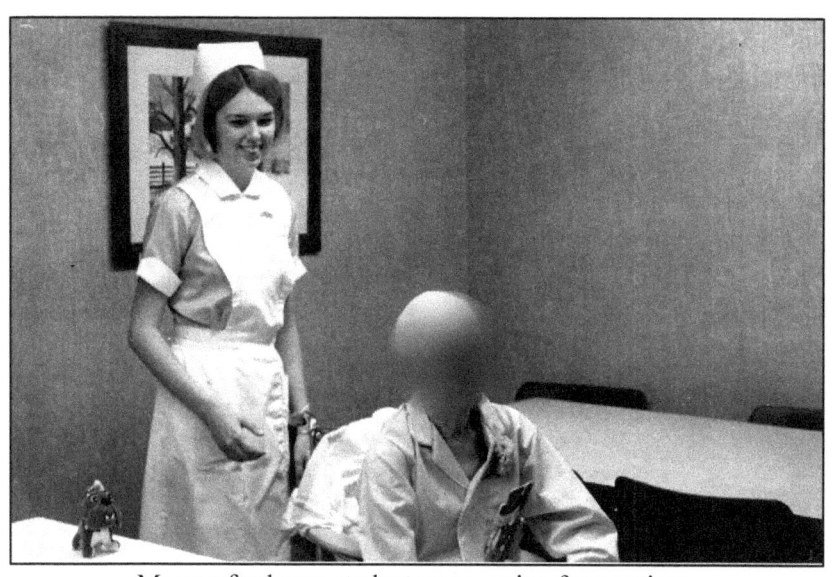
Me as a freshman student nurse caring for a patient

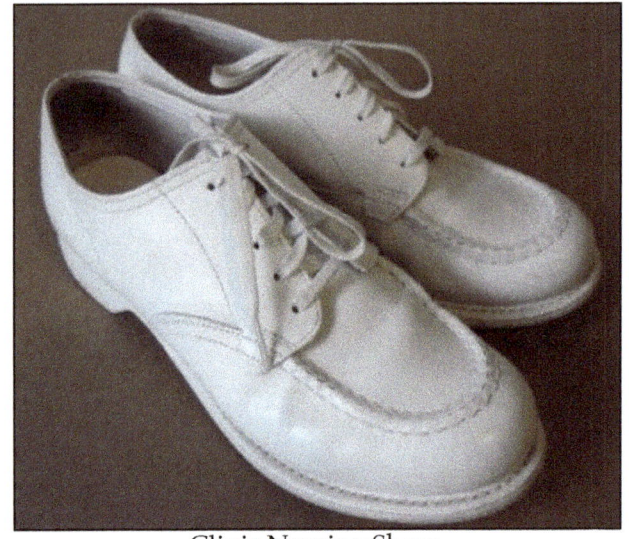
Clinic Nursing Shoes

My student ID from summer school 1969

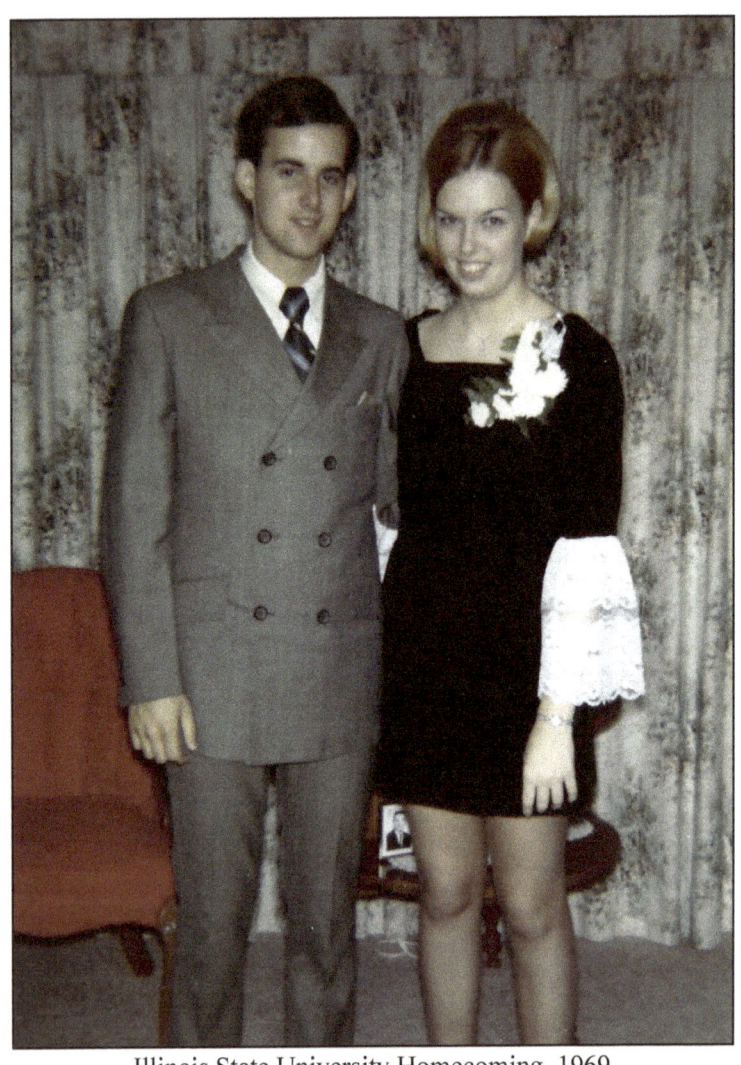
Illinois State University Homecoming, 1969

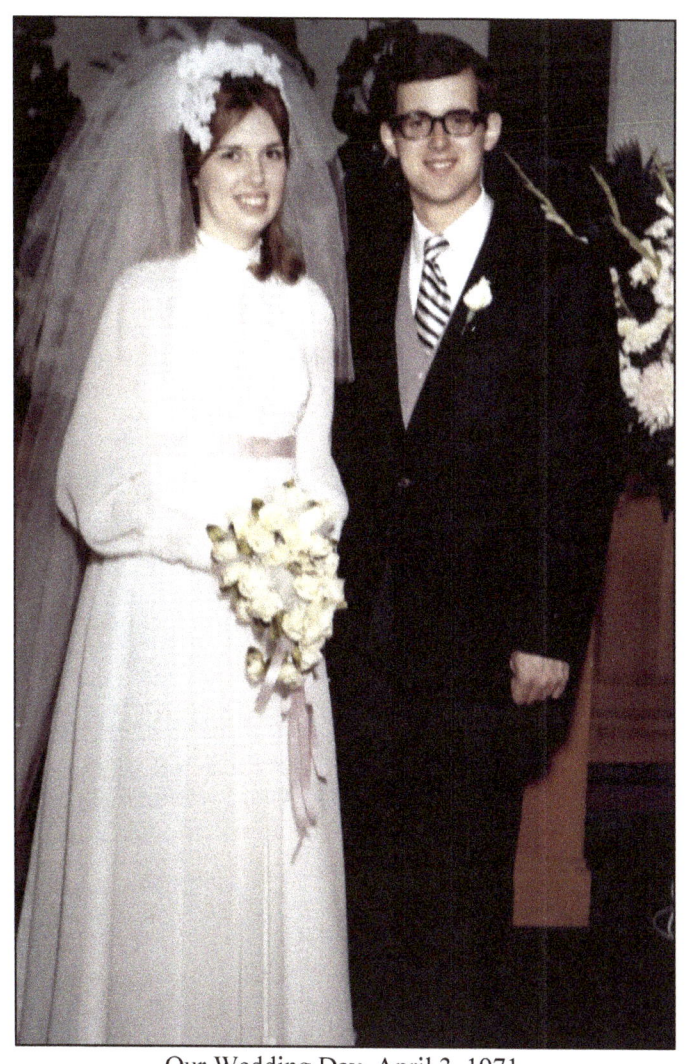
Our Wedding Day, April 3, 1971

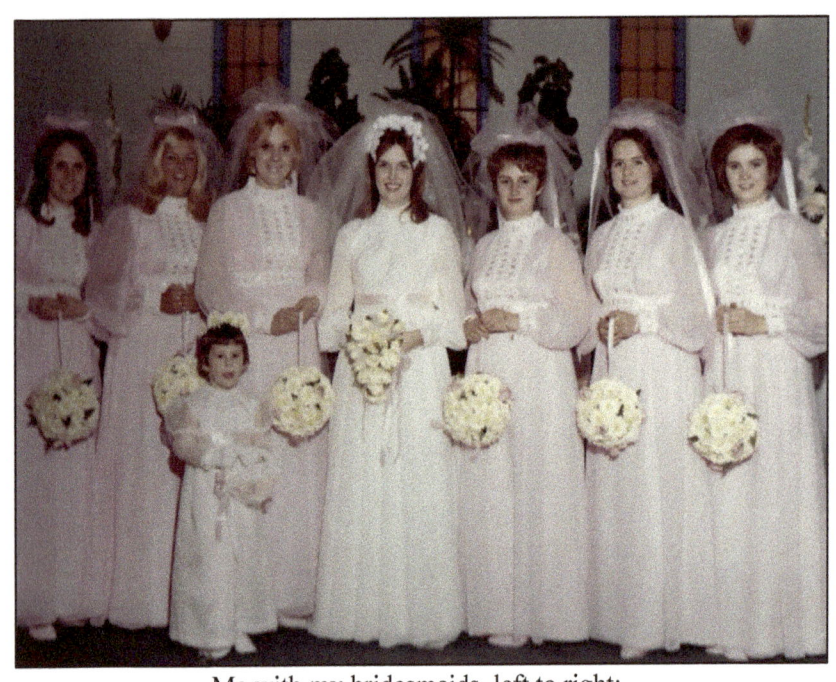

Me with my bridesmaids, left to right:
my roommate freshman and junior years, Cynthia,
Kay Beth, me, sister-in-law SanDee, sister-in-law Linda,
my cousin Barb, my cousin Angie as flower girl

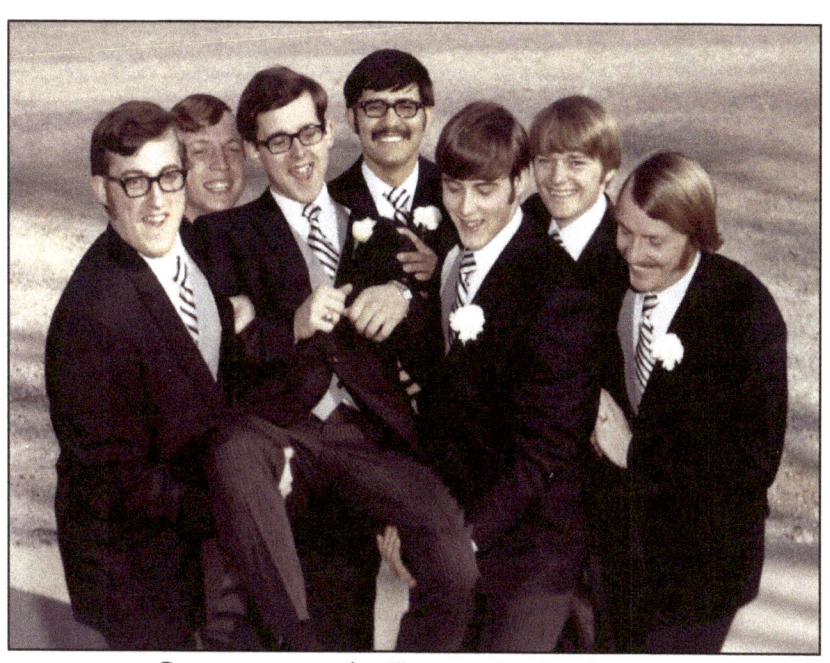
Groomsmen carrying Terry up the church steps

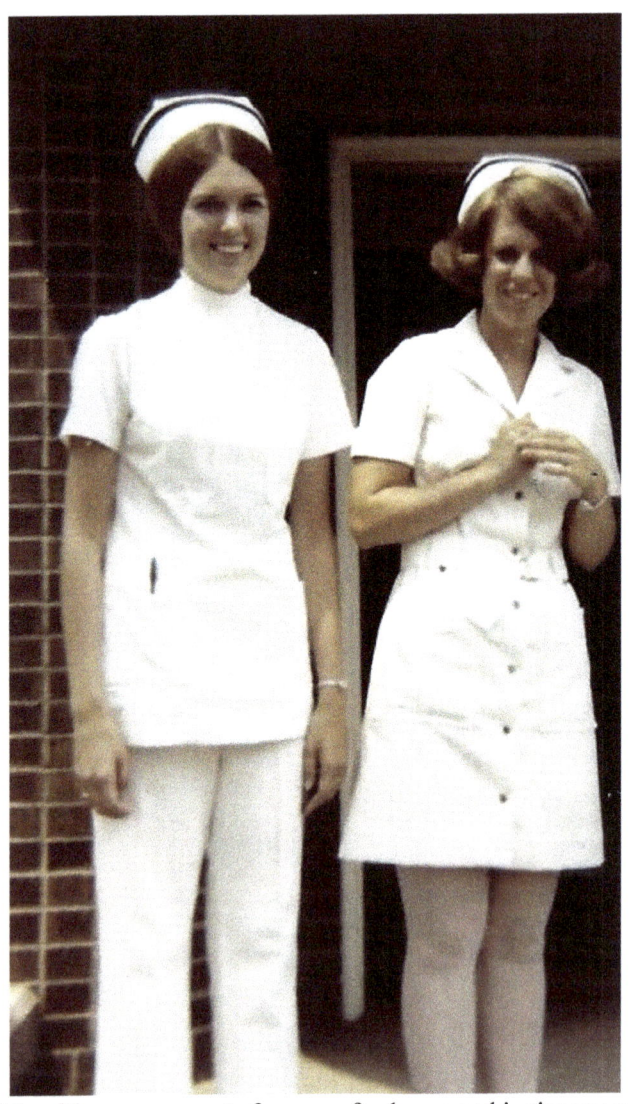

Me with my roommate from my freshman and junior years on our last day of school

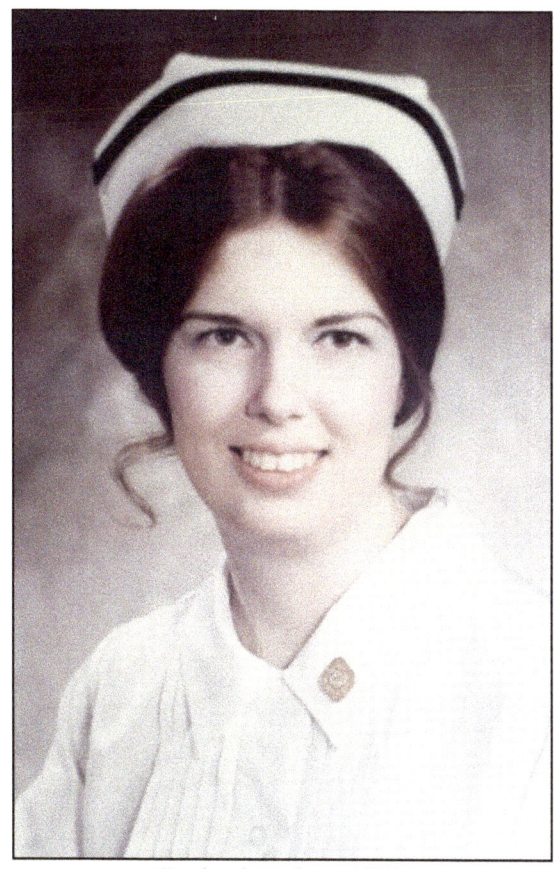
Graduation photo 1971

# Program

Organ Prelude ..................................................... Mrs. Marcia Hishman

*Processional—Psalm XVIX ................................................ Marcello

*Invocation ........................................................... William E. Dunn
  Chairman, School of Nursing Board
  Executive Vice-President, Mennonite Hospital

Hymn—Now Thank We All Our God ........................................ No. 49
  (Congregation Join in Singing)

Scripture ....................................................... John C. Stutzman, M.D.
  Member, School of Nursing Board

Address—People Need People .................................. Richard G. Watts
  Minister, First United Presbyterian Church
  Normal, Illinois

Remarks ............................................................... William E. Dunn

Introduction of Graduating Class ......................... Mrs. Louise Watson
  Faculty Advisor

Presentation of Diplomas ........................................... William E. Dunn

Presentation of Pins ................................... Mrs. Jacquelyn S. Kinder
  Director, School of Nursing

Anthem—From These Halls ........................................... Haydn-McLin
  Graduating Class
  Ronald D. Ropp, Director

*Benediction ...................................................... Miss Lora Rentfro

*Recessional—Psalm XX .................................................. Marcello

*Congregation Standing

Reception follows in the Lower Fellowship Hall

Program from my commencement

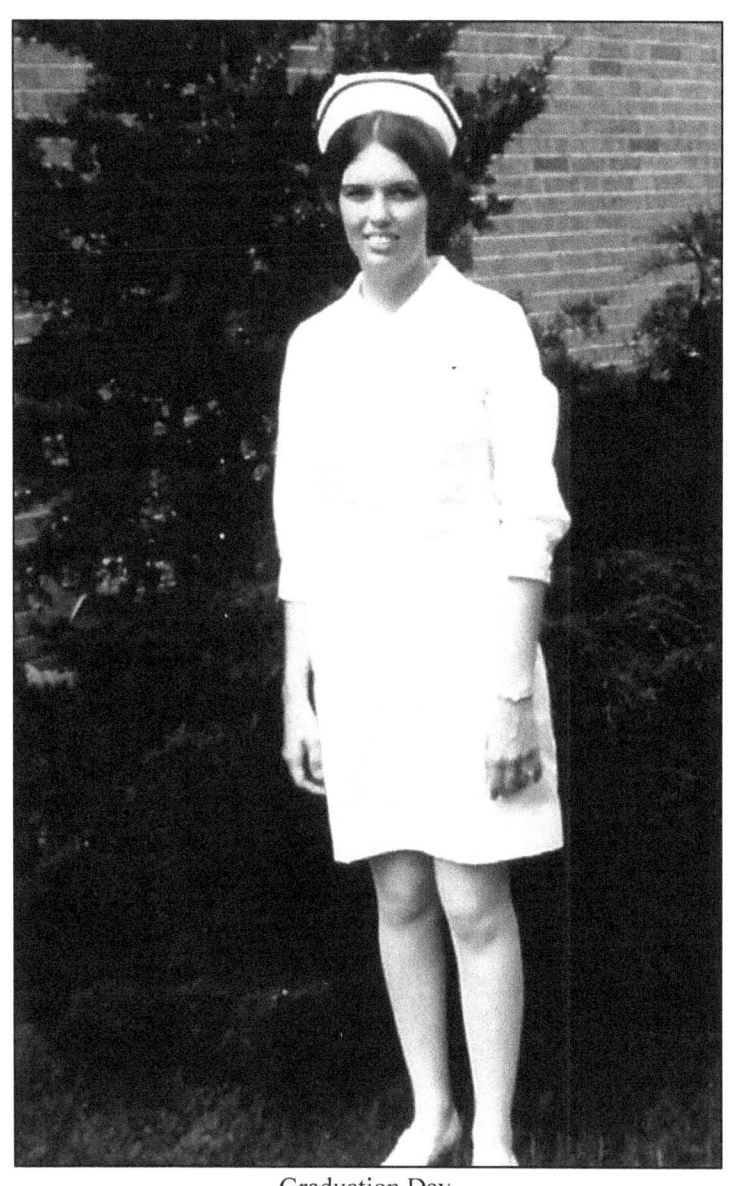
Graduation Day

# Mennonite Hospital School of Nursing

**Bloomington, Illinois**

This Certifies That

### Ila M. Minnick

has completed the required course of instruction in the theory and practice of nursing and having passed the required examinations is awarded this

**Diploma**

Given at Bloomington, in the State of Illinois,
June 20, 1971.

*Jacquelyn S. Kinder, R.N.*
Director, School of Nursing

*William E. Dunn*
Chairman, School of Nursing Board

My Nursing Diploma

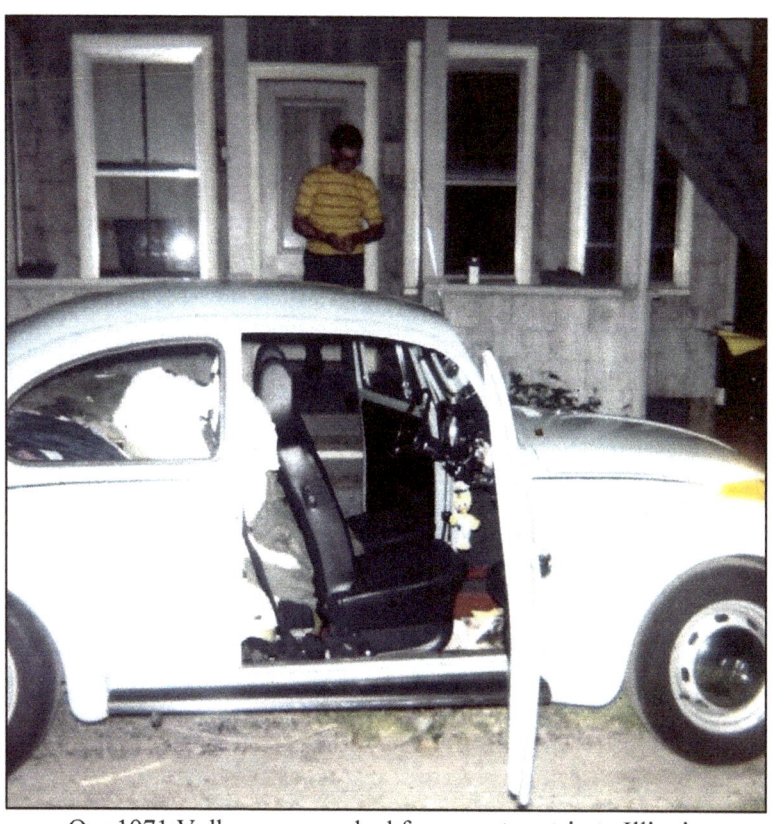
Our 1971 Volkswagen packed for our return trip to Illinois

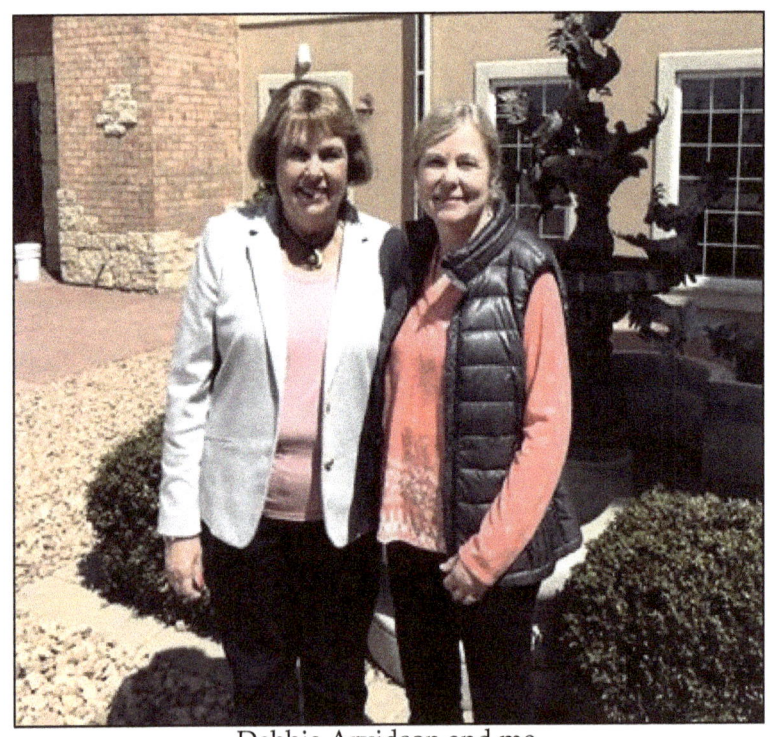
Debbie Arvidson and me

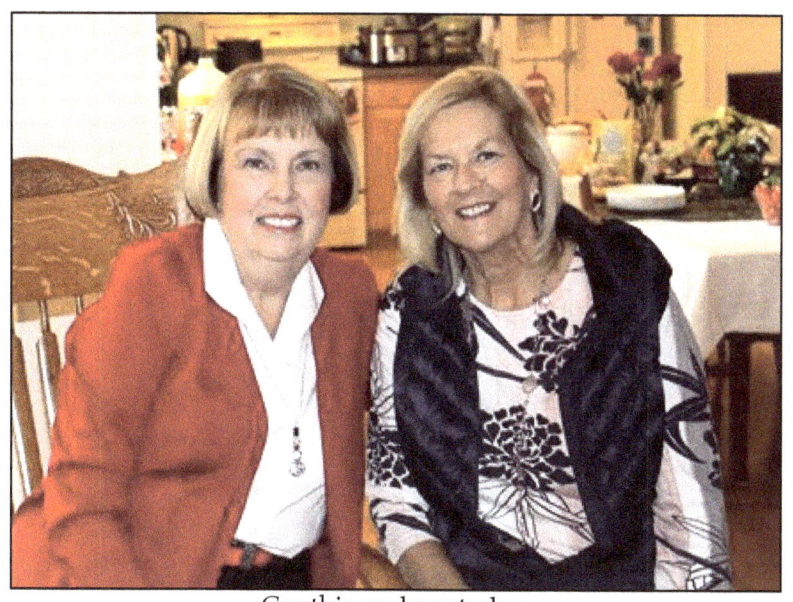
Cynthia and me today

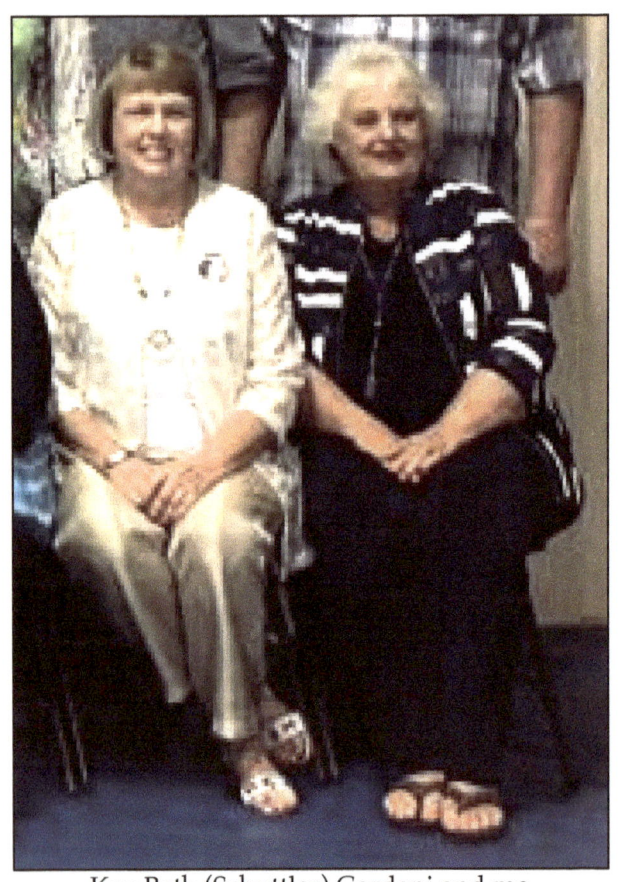

Kay Beth (Schuttler) Cordani and me
at our 50th high school class reunion in 2018.
Kay Beth died in 2024.

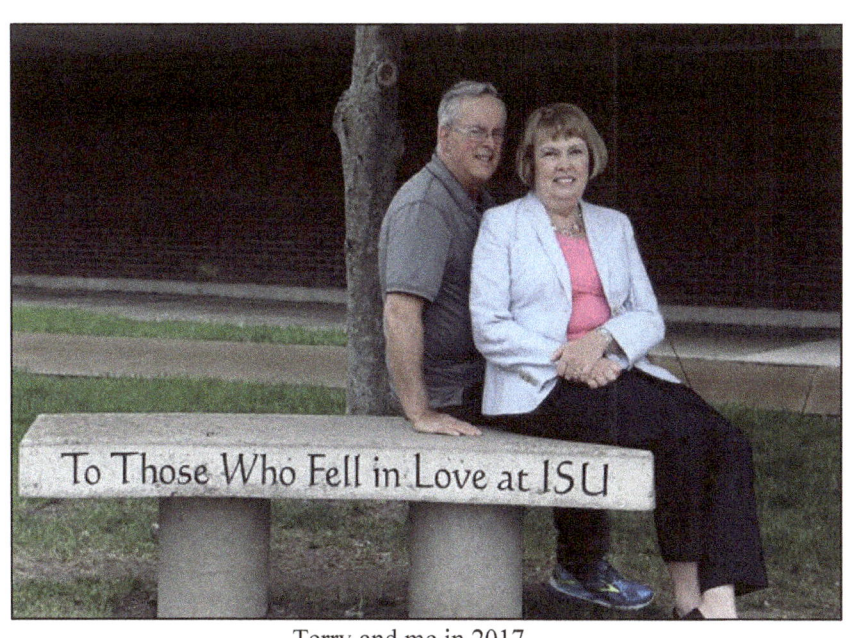

Terry and me in 2017,
on the
"To Those who Fell in Love at ISU" bench

# 5

## Junior Year 1969 – 1970

*Proverbs 3:5, 6 Trust in the Lord with all your heart, and do not lean on your own understanding. In all your ways acknowledge him, and he will direct your paths.*

Junior year meant I was now an upperclassman and more confident about my place in school and clinicals. I enjoyed a great roommate while cultivating wonderful friendships with fellow nursing students. I had developed my rhythm, so to speak. With the required ISU college courses completed, the coursework would now focus on nursing and increasingly complex clinical skills. Our clinical time increased to 16 hours a week – I do not recall how that was divided, but it was at least 4 hours a day.

I continued spending most weekends at Illinois State University with Kay Beth Schuttler, a close high school friend. I often hopped on the city bus on Friday afternoon, heading to ISU, then took a cab or walked the three miles on my return trip on Sunday, as the buses did not run on Sundays. I was grateful for the time away from the quiet, deserted nursing dorm. I am sure we shared many laughs and secrets in her little dorm room and provided ongoing aggravation for her roommate.

Terry and I continued dating through my junior year. When Terry picked me up at Mennonite, I often waited by the door until he pulled up in his mint green 1963 Volkswagen Beetle. I would run down the steps, hop into the car, and off we'd go. On other occasions, I heard the housemother announce, "Ila Ethell, you have a visitor in the lobby". We enjoyed many adventures in that little car. He taught me to drive a "stick shift," resulting in that poor little car enduring much jerking and pitching. We made trips to Springfield, Rockford, Manito, Peoria, and other Illinois destinations. Miller Park in Bloomington, with its beautiful lake and little zoo, was a favorite destination in nice weather.

Terry lived with four other guys in an apartment in a professor's home at 601 N. Main in Normal. It was affectionately known as 601. We frequently purchased a 25-cent box of Kraft spaghetti mix and a 6-oz can of tomato paste to prepare a delicious spaghetti dinner on the hot plate in their living area. Because they only had one hot plate and one pan, we cooked the spaghetti first, then the sauce. When the street was widened many years later, the house was torn down.

McDonald's was a frequent stop, as was Pizza Hut, Lum's restaurant, and of course Normal's iconic Tobin's Pizza. For homecoming or special occasions, we went to Sinorak, the big Smorgasbord in Bloomington. We thought that was a real treat. Brandtville Truck Stop was also a favorite place as they were open all night and known for their fried chicken. It was common to find the place hopping with college students after everything else had closed.

He invited me to Rockford, where we spent time with his family, met his high school friends, and visited his old haunts. We enjoyed the Top Hat Restaurant in Loves Park, Illinois, with their large buffet and complimentary home-baked loaf of bread, strawberry pie at the Hollywood

Restaurant, and viewing movies at one of the local theatres. Butch Cassidy and the Sundance Kid was a favorite. I also recall seeing Goodbye Columbus (I was so naïve, I didn't understand the title), The Graduate, MASH, and Love Story. I loved attending his church with its beautiful music and Bible-centered sermons. I had never participated in a church quite like it, and I enjoyed it so much.

## Obstetrics and Gynecology

My junior year began with Obstetrics and Gynecology (now called Maternal-Child Health). The prospect of seeing an actual birth was exciting to me. Our clinical rotation consisted of Labor and Delivery, Post-Partum, and the newborn nursery.

Giving birth in a hospital differed from today's practice. Birthing rooms did not exist, and babies were born in delivery rooms with an obstetrician in attendance. Midwives did not practice in hospitals and were less prevalent or autonomous than they are today. The preparation for delivery was more intrusive, requiring the mother to endure a more extensive perineal shave and a soap suds enema. It must have been so uncomfortable for the laboring woman to receive a complete enema during their pain. Fathers were usually, but not always, present in the labor rooms with their wives.

The Lamaze method of childbirth was taught, but was inconsistently utilized. Women unfamiliar with Lamaze were coached to use effleurage, where the woman made light, round, circular motions around her abdomen to focus and calm her. My observations led me to conclude that this was an ineffective method of coping with labor. Although epidurals and saddle blocks were available, I did not see them used during my rotation.

Penthrane anesthetic gas was frequently used to dull the pain and consciousness during labor. Liquid Penthrane was poured into a round cylinder with an attached black rubber mask used for inhalation. As the discomfort intensified, the patient was instructed to inhale the anesthetic vapor through the black rubber mask. The patient did not experience general anesthesia but was less conscious and somewhat more comfortable. As an anesthetic gas, Penthrane had a pungent smell, so the laboring woman might be reluctant to use it after one or two whiffs. With no epidural or effective pain control, labor and delivery units were noisier than the present day, as the laboring women cried out in agony from the intense pain.

Mothers gave birth in the delivery room, necessitating transfer from the labor room to the delivery room, a bright, sterile environment with stainless steel stirrups, a large overhead light, and stainless-steel tables. It resembled an operating room rather than a warm and friendly birthing room. Fathers did NOT accompany their wives in the delivery room, preventing them from seeing their new son or daughter until after the birth was complete and someone brought the baby to them. They did not share the moment of birth as a couple or family. The father often met the baby away from his wife. Overall, it was a less personalized experience for the family.

Women remained in the hospital for about five days following a vaginal birth and seven to 10 days following a Cesarean Section. During the post-partum clinical, we cared for the new mothers following the birth of their babies. Because assessment and observation are fundamental components of nursing care, we developed the required skills for this rotation. We learned to palpate the top of the uterus, or fundus, to check the size and consistency of the uterus as it contracted and began returning to normal size. Following delivery, the uterus should contract one centimeter (.394 inches) every 24 hours and return to its normal size and location within the pelvis by six weeks. We monitored the lochia or post-birth discharge, assessing for hemorrhage and infection. We assisted with the required education for breastfeeding the newborn and monitored the mother for signs of an infection.

Rooming in, where the baby stayed in the mother's room, was uncommon. Most babies remained in the newborn nursery and were brought to the mother at regular intervals for feeding and bonding. Therefore, we also cared for the babies by learning to feed, burp, diaper, bathe, clothe, and swaddle them in a blanket. We sometimes observed circumcision on male babies.

Children under 12 were not allowed to visit, so younger siblings could only view their new brother or sister through the nursery window. They did not interact with the baby until their mother and sibling were discharged. Although breastfeeding was an option, it was not enthusiastically encouraged, making formula-fed babies the norm.

This rotation provided the opportunity to be paired with expectant mothers, who allowed us to "follow" them through their entire birthing experience. We accompanied them to some of their obstetrical appointments before and after the baby was born. We were attentive as the obstetrician monitored her progress before the baby's arrival and following birth. In addition to the obstetrician appointments, I recall accompanying my mom and her baby to one of their pediatrician appointments following the baby's birth. I was fortunate to be paired with a nurse who, with her husband, welcomed my participation in their birthing experience. As her time of delivery drew near, I was "on call" to accompany her to the hospital when she went into active labor. I recall that this occurred for my patient around 11 PM. A taxi transported me to the hospital, where I remained with the patient and her husband all night until their baby girl was born the next morning. I participated in her preparation, assisted her and her husband with Lamaze, and was present for the delivery. I accompanied her to the recovery area and cared for her in the post-partum unit. I visited the family at home several weeks after discharge. This family welcomed me into their lives, and I visited them throughout my time in nursing school. They sent me pictures and cards, and we stayed in touch for a while after I graduated from Mennonite. It is amazing to think that the baby is now in her 50s.

**Self-Care Unit**

Expensive, high-tech diagnostic tools were not yet available. Computed tomography (CT) scanners were first used in 1972, and most hospitals did not yet own one (Kumar, 2023). Highly sophisticated Magnetic Resonance Imaging (MRI) technology was not utilized until 1977 (Garet, 2020). Therefore, Mennonite Hospital owned neither of these imaging machines during my time there. Today, the necessary information is often obtained from ONE test, such as a CT scan, ultrasound, PET scan, or MRI. The lack of current technology meant patients underwent multiple tests such as barium enema, barium swallow, intravenous pyelogram, myelogram, sigmoidoscopy, and lumbar puncture to obtain a diagnosis. Many of these tests were uncomfortable, painful, and might require unpleasant preparations.

Mennonite utilized a self-care unit where patients who could care for themselves were admitted for "testing" and remained in the hospital for several days until their diagnostic tests were completed. The nursing staff oversaw preparations for any tests the patient underwent, eliminating the need for patient guesswork. A bowel prep might require the patient to receive oral castor oil to clear the colon, followed by repeated enemas until the water was expelled clear. Oral medication might be administered the night before the exam. Food and water were usually withheld after midnight before the test. The nursing staff assumed responsibility for completing all preparations as ordered, while observing the patient's response to these exhausting preparations.

Spending time on this unit allowed the student nurse to learn about the various medical tests, x-rays, and bloodwork the patients underwent, and the disease process the doctor could be looking for. After reviewing the patient's chart and spending time with them discussing their symptoms and history, we assimilated all the information to correlate the purpose of the tests with our research. We provided the necessary care once the tests were completed and often learned the results of the tests. Because the patients weren't technically "sick", we could spend time talking with them and discussing their overall health. We identified lifestyle changes the patient might need to pursue and provided education to contribute to their successful changes. Although we provided minimal hands-on care, the time spent on that unit was a valuable learning opportunity.

## Pediatrics

While prior classes traveled to and lived in Chicago for this rotation, we were the first class to avoid spending a six-week Pediatric rotation at Children's Memorial Hospital in Chicago, Illinois. We received our Pediatric clinical experience at St. Joseph's, a local Catholic community hospital in Bloomington, Illinois. The rationale was that we would observe the more common childhood diseases locally. Children's Memorial provided experience for the sickest children with high acuity and uncommon diseases not experienced every day. I was not sorry to miss living in Chicago for the six-week Pediatric rotation.

Of interest, the pediatric clinical experience at St. Joseph's Hospital adhered to an interesting medical hierarchy practice. My nursing education occurred shortly after the era when nurses were expected to relinquish their chairs when a doctor entered the unit. In other words, if a nurse was seated at the nurse's station, most likely working, and a doctor entered the unit, the nurse was expected to stop what he/she was doing, get up from their seat, and offer that seat to the physician. This followed a strict medical hierarchy common throughout the 1960s. By the 1970s, this practice was beginning to wane. However, in 1969, St. Joseph's Hospital, site of my pediatric clinical experience, still held to that practice. Any nurse, and most certainly a student nurse, seated at the nurse's station rose and gave up her chair to the doctor when he arrived.

As students, we cared for many children experiencing pediatric illnesses. Dehydration due to a gastrointestinal virus was a common cause of admission. Because children experience dehydration much faster than adults, we quickly learned how to assess the child for signs of dehydration. Rather than always starting an intravenous infusion (IV) to replace fluids as we do today, hypodermoclysis was a frequent treatment for fluid and electrolyte replacement. Although the treatment was common practice for pediatric patients, today this treatment modality may be used to treat frail elderly patients requiring fluids. The procedure consisted of inserting a long (approximately 2-inch) needle into each of the child's thighs, taping it in place, and slowly infusing the fluid. The child was restrained so they did not inadvertently or purposely interfere with the treatment. My heart went out to these children, and even now, I cringe thinking about it. The treatment looked uncomfortable, and it must have been so painful and frightening when those needles were inserted.

Although meningitis was fairly uncommon, when it was suspected, we assisted with the diagnostic lumbar puncture by setting up for the procedure and holding the child in the correct position. For this procedure, the doctor inserted a needle between the lumbar vertebrae into the spinal column to withdraw spinal fluid to determine the presence of bacteria and signs of infection. The patient was curled in a ball with the knees as close to the chest as possible to separate the bony vertebrae and allow access into the spinal meninges. The test was terrifying to the little patients, and there were times when we shed tears with them.

It was during my pediatric rotation that I observed my first operation, an appendectomy on a 12-year-old boy. When it was decided that the boy required surgery, my classmate and I requested to remain past our scheduled shift to observe it. I recall the kind staff providing surgical attire, instructing us how to wear the cap and mask, where to stand, and what to avoid while in the operating room. We greeted our young patient when he entered so he would know that familiar faces were with him. Following the general anesthesia induction, the surgeon was gowned and gloved, the skin was prepped, surgical drapes were placed, and the necessary instruments and equipment were arranged around the patient. The surgeon adjusted the bright lights over the surgical site, and the operation began. I think because I had looked forward to observing surgery, I was not the least bit queasy. Having never stood in such surroundings, I was fascinated with the whole scene as I looked around the room, taking it all in. We watched intently as the surgeon incised the skin and dissected the abdominal tissues to locate and remove the appendix. Before the specimen was sent to the lab, the surgeon explained the appearance of the infected appendix compared to a normal appendix. I cared for the patient during his hospital stay and found it interesting to follow him from diagnosis to discharge.

To provide a robust learning experience, we visited several community organizations. The most memorable visit was to a children's home, which provided long-term care for severely physically and emotionally challenged children. I recall walking into the large pediatric ward, where rows of metal cribs held children, many of them suffering from hydrocephalus, a condition caused by a blocked brain ventricle that prevents cerebrospinal fluid from draining properly. The excess cerebrospinal fluid caused their skull to expand, resulting in their heads being disproportionate in size and weight to their bodies. Retention of the cerebrospinal fluid made their heads heavy, preventing them from voluntarily lifting their heads from the bed. Their heads had to be cautiously supported during feeding or other activities. Today's technology provides a better outcome for these children. Although hydrocephalus still exists, children can live mostly normal lives after having the fluid shunted and drained from their heads.

**Surgery**

As a preface to my Operating Room (OR) educational experience, let me point out that schools of nursing eventually removed the OR from nursing curricula. Although I am unaware of the exact timeframe for that decision, I know that the OR nursing education experience was phased out. At my first place of employment, which had a diploma school, the Perioperative Nursing rotation was eight weeks long, with four weeks spent in the OR and four weeks in the Recovery Room (RR), currently called the Post Anesthesia Care Unit (PACU). This organization discontinued the Perioperative Nursing course around 1978. Consider that the only way nursing students or a registered nurse will know if she/he would like to work in the operating room is by first-hand experience. Many surgical departments are searching for experienced nurses to staff and lead their departments. OR nursing leaders are retiring, but there is a shortage of qualified people to take their place. I will provide additional details in my next book. But that is a story for a different day.

Guided by research and evidence-based standards established by the professional organization, the Association of periOperative Registered Nurses (AORN), nurses maintain constant vigilance in monitoring the OR environment before, during and after surgery. This relentless vigilance allows patients to safely undergo surgical procedures. AORN standards direct all aspects of nursing care in the operating room, preoperatively (before the operation), intraoperatively (during the operation), and postoperatively (after the operation). These standards apply to many aspects of the patient experience but are taught most succinctly in the operating room.

OR nursing practice epitomizes precision, organization, and surgical conscience. Precision means that everything is done a certain way without deviation. Organization means every step is executed in an orderly, prescribed way to accomplish the work in a tight timeframe with unwavering attention to patient safety. Surgical conscience means we do the right thing and adhere to strict guidelines at all times because the health of our patients depends on it. It holds each member of the surgical team accountable for any breach in safety or aseptic technique. Surgical conscience instills the importance of each individual assuming responsibility and rectifying compromise, whether or not anyone is looking.

The practice of sterile technique, also known as asepsis or aseptic technique is hardwired in the OR. No area outside of the OR provides the principles of aseptic technique or demands adherence to those principles like the OR. Asepsis creates an environment that drastically reduces the impact of germs and bacteria on the patient during the surgical procedure. While today's nursing students are taught aseptic technique, the strictest aseptic technique is best learned in the OR. Aseptic technique establishes what is sterile and not sterile, and is key to guarding patients from life-threatening infections. The OR teaches the principles of disinfection, clean vs dirty, disinfected vs sterile, and all-important principles to keep patients safe during surgical procedures. Isla Stewart said, "The success of the surgical nurse of the present day depends entirely on her ability to understand and appreciate the theory of 'asepsis', or surgical cleanliness, which underlies the practice of modern surgery, and her capacity for intelligent attention to the minutest detail" (Hallet, 2010, p. 93). Of note, nurses are only referred to as female because, at that time, nursing was a female-dominated profession, and physicians were a male-dominated profession.

After those introductory statements, I return to my student experience. It was finally time for my Operating Room (OR) rotation, and I was more than ready. Excitement was the word of the day as I attained the opportunity to participate in surgical procedures. I didn't care about the level of my participation; just let me in there! To provide a robust learning experience, our class was divided into smaller groups to scrub and circulate cases with our preceptors. As I recall, Mennonite's OR suite consisted of one major room, two minor rooms, and a Urology room. Sterile supplies and anesthesia equipment were also housed within the OR suite.

The first thing one must learn about the surgical suite is how to navigate it. In other words, what to do once I get in the door, adherence to proper attire including what do I wear and when do I wear it, where can I go, where am I not allowed to go, where do I stand, what can I touch, not touch, and if I am not scrubbed at the field, how do I get close enough to visualize the procedure without contaminating the entire surgical field?

The OR department is divided into three zones: unrestricted, semi-restricted, and restricted. Surgical departments are designed to accommodate these traffic patterns. The unrestricted area permits street clothes and scrub attire. It usually includes the control area of the department, locker rooms, the Preoperative preparation area, and the Recovery Room. The Semi-restricted area requires the wearing of scrub attire, but masks are not required. Street clothes are not permitted here. The restricted area is anywhere there are open sterile items inside the operating room itself, necessitating all personnel to wear masks. The very foreign environment and our novice state led to some anxiety on our part. In addition, some surgeons had a reputation for being gruff with staff, heightening our fear of making mistakes and incurring the surgeon's ire.

All activity in the OR has a prescribed way of getting accomplished. To lessen the stirring up of dust and bacteria, there is an established traffic flow for the department and the individual operating room. The goal is to keep the sterile field sterile to minimize the risk of infection for the patient. The furnishings that will hold the sterile supplies are arranged in a precise way. The sterile supplies are set up and opened in a certain order to prevent contamination. When dispensing something onto the sterile field, if a single part is contaminated, the whole field may be compromised, forcing one to start over. This provides some insight as to why we were terrified. And although it has happened to me on numerous occasions, no one wants to be the reason an entire surgical setup gets contaminated. Starting over costs time and surgeon patience, resulting in embarrassment. However, surgical conscience dictates that we do the right thing and address errors honestly, so embarrassment is never a reason to compromise patient safety.

For this rotation, students were assigned only to the operating room. Later in our education, we would "follow" a patient, which meant preparing the patient for surgery, accompanying him or her to the operating room, observing the surgery, and caring for the patient post-operatively. As preparation for our time in the operating room, we reviewed the OR schedule the night before, studied the surgical procedures, and researched the patient's diagnosis that warranted the surgery.

One of the first things we learned was the proper procedure for scrubbing our hands and donning the sterile gown and gloves. The surgical scrub is a meticulous process with steps completed in order and in a prescribed way according to standards. While the hands cannot be sterilized or scrubbed free from all germs, the goal is to reduce as much bacteria on the skin as possible.

Before scrubbing our hands, we selected our sterile gown and the correct size gloves and opened them on the mayo stand, the mobile stand that would eventually hold the instruments required "at the ready" during the procedure. We proceeded to the "scrub sink" and began by washing our hands and arms with soap and water. Our attention was laser-focused on the faucet and sink area because once we started the scrub, we couldn't touch anything. Not watching where our hands were risked inadvertently touching the faucet, requiring us to restart the surgical scrub. Because we could not touch the soap dispenser or use our hands to adjust the faucet, soap was dispensed by operating a foot pump, and water was dispensed by activating a switch with our knees. Frustration and embarrassment would ensue if we had to start over.

Each scrub sink was stocked with two types of brushes. Stiff bristled brushes were used for scrubbing the fingernails, fingers, and hands. Softer bristled brushes were used to scrub the entire arm. The brush package contained a nail file for thoroughly cleaning our fingernails under running water. The initial surgical scrub each morning was required to last ten minutes, which we timed using the clock. Subsequent hand scrubs were five minutes unless we were scrubbing for orthopedic surgery, which required a ten-minute scrub for each case. The surgical scrub began by washing the hands with soap and water and cleaning fingernails with the file. Using the stiff-bristled brush filled with soap, the fingernails and tips of the fingers were scrubbed 20 strokes. Continuing with the stiff-bristled brush, fingers were scrubbed by dividing each finger's surface into four sections and scrubbing each section 20 strokes. Each area of the hand, including the wrist, was scrubbed 20 strokes. Once the hands were scrubbed, they were rinsed starting with the fingers and then the hand, allowing the water to run downward toward the elbow to avoid contaminating the hands with water dripping from the arms which were not yet scrubbed. We were mindful of the faucet because it was easy to inadvertently touch it as our hands were brought upward through the running water. None of us got through this rotation without touching something and repeating the scrub. We quickly learned to be careful and deliberate to avoid this embarrassment and waste of valuable time. Because hard bristles were painful on more sensitive skin areas, arms were scrubbed using the softer-bristle brush. Each surface of the arm was scrubbed for ten strokes, including halfway up the upper arm. Then the hands and arms were rinsed in the same manner, allowing the water to run down over the elbow to avoid contaminating the hands. The student was then ready to enter the operating room and don the gown and gloves.

Again, there was a prescribed way to do this to avoid contaminating things. Interestingly, we were taught a closed gloving technique, where the hands did not go through the gown's cuff. The gloves were donned while our hands remained inside the gown sleeves. Until the technique is mastered, it is very awkward and prone to mistakes. As students, we endured our share of flubs and "do-overs".

Next came the case set-up, where we organized everything on the back table and arranged the instruments. Instruments to be used immediately were arranged in the order they would be used and were readily available on the Mayo stand. Everything else remained on the back table. Different sutures (stitching material) were used for various stages of the surgical wound closure and were arranged accordingly. Before beginning the operation, sponges and possibly instruments were counted. Current practice requires that many more items be counted. If a body cavity such as the abdomen or chest is opened, nearly everything on the field is counted – sponges, needles, scalpel blades, all instruments, cautery blades, cautery cleaning pad, and screws present on some of the retractors.

While the majority of today's surgical supplies are disposable and intended for one-time use, formerly everything was cloth and/or reusable. Surgical drapes, sponges used in the abdomen, towels, some syringes, basins, and many other items were all reused. This required manpower for washing, drying, wrapping, preparing for sterilization, sterilizing everything, and restocking the shelves for the next day's cases. Today's disposable surgical supplies require less manpower and fewer steps.

We worked primarily with several general surgeons and a urologist. Mennonite Hospital performed minimal orthopedic procedures and no obstetrics or gynecological procedures. I recall one of the general surgeons bowing his head and praying before he began the procedure. After he entered the operating room and donned his gown and gloves, he paused to pray. This impressed me because I knew he was offering himself as God's servant by uniting his hands with the hands of God and asking for wisdom to do the right thing for the patient. The other surgeon had a private scrub nurse who worked with him in the office, accompanied him on hospital rounds, and assisted him in surgery. They intimidated me, not because they were mean, but because they worked as a no-nonsense team aware of each other's moves with minimal conversation required. The surgeon could be gruff, which was intimidating to a 19-year-old woman. I also recall a dentist giving the anesthetic for a tonsillectomy. Dentists were some of the first anesthesia providers.

I loved this rotation with the surgical nurses who taught us and provided opportunities to scrub and circulate the surgical cases with them. The surgical team consisted of the surgeon, the assistant, the anesthesia provider who would be an anesthetist (RN trained in anesthesia administration) or an anesthesiologist (MD specializing in anesthesia), the scrub nurse, and the circulating nurse.

The scrub nurse can be a Surgical Technologist or an RN. They stand in the operative field next to the surgeon, monitor the procedure, understand where the surgeon is in the procedure, and anticipate the next thing he/she will need. They hand the instruments, prepare sutures, handle any specimens until the surgeon permits them to be handed off the sterile field, and ensure all necessary sterile supplies are available and ready. Because they are part of the "sterile field", they remain at the OR table and can only touch items in the sterile field. The circulating nurse provides all sterile items to the scrub nurse.

The circulating nurse must be a Registered Nurse. She/he coordinates all activities in the operating room and is responsible for the patient's nursing care. The circulating nurse "circulates" the room with attention to all room activities and the patient's status. She/he ensures that everything is ready for each patient's surgery by reviewing the patient's chart, making sure all documents are present and appropriately signed, and interviewing the patient to identify and mitigate potential issues. In partnership with the scrub nurse, the circulating nurse reviews the surgeon's instruments, supplies, and procedural preferences, making sure the correct equipment is in the room and safely functioning. She/he brings the patient into the operating room, helps settle the patient on the OR bed, and supports the anesthesia provider. The circulating nurse assists the anesthetist or anesthesiologist by remaining at the patient's side until the induction of anesthesia is complete. She/he helps position and prepare the patient's operative site with constant vigilance for adherence to sterile technique and other safety measures. The circulating nurse is responsible for operating all equipment that the procedure requires. Once the procedure is underway, the circulating nurse completes the necessary paperwork, including charting on the medical record, charging for supplies, and handling specimens. Those nurses observe the operative field to anticipate the next steps. When wound closure begins, the circulating nurse oversees counting items that could be retained in the patient's body. She/he communicates the patient's status with other departments such as PACU, Laboratory, and the OR control area to ensure subsequent patients are sent for at the appropriate time.

**Summer School, 1970**

Following my junior year, I again enrolled in summer school at ISU to obtain additional college credits. Having remained in contact with a friend from the prior year's summer school experience, she and I decided to room together. She was a delightful girl, and we located a very nice apartment in the home of a retired female Army

Lieutenant Colonel. Her large home contained several apartment living spaces, each with three bedrooms, a bathroom, a kitchen, and a community living area. It was located close to campus, and I enjoyed living there. There was no need to worry about security because the Lieutenant Colonel ran a very tight ship. With no dorm cafeteria, we were responsible for our meals. My roommate was a great cook and taught me how to make several dishes, including cheese sauce. I have used her cheese sauce recipe since then.

Not having a car meant walking or relying on other transportation. One night we decided to order a pizza and about 11 p.m., one of my suite mates and I set out on foot to pick it up a few blocks away. Delivery was not always an option, as not every pizza place delivered. As we were walking along the campus perimeter, a carload of guys pulled up alongside us and began harassing us. The carload of guys was on one side of us with a tall chain link fence on the other side, eliminating any opportunity for escape. My first response was to ignore them, but my friend warned me it would only worsen the situation. We politely engaged with them as they drove slowly beside us and continued harassing us. They finally drove away, leaving both of us pretty shaken. This would not be my last encounter with a potentially dangerous situation.

I enjoyed the English Literature and Political Science courses I anticipated would be required if I returned to school. It was fun spending time with people other than nursing students and learning something besides nursing. The huge political science classroom helped validate that I was a very small fish in a large pond.

Terry had graduated from ISU in June and enlisted in the Army in July. After spending so much time together during his senior year at ISU, we had to adjust to long separation intervals. He left for basic training at Fort Leonard Wood, Missouri on July 29, 1970. I rode the bus from Bloomington, Illinois to Rockford to see him off. The return ride to school was a pretty lonely bus ride. His first letter arrived at my home in Manito, and after learning that I had a letter waiting for me, I asked if my parents could bring it to me. My dad got in the car, drove the 45 minutes to Normal, and brought the letter to me after we hung up. I was so happy to receive it.

Before long, it was time to return to school for my senior year! Two years had flown by, and now all of my classes would take place at the school of nursing with increasing clinical hours.

# 6

## Senior Year 1970-1971

*Commit your work to the Lord, and your plans will be established. Proverbs 16:3*

Because my roommate married after our junior year, I elected not to live in the dorm my senior year. I joined two other nursing students as we shared a two-bedroom apartment with three ISU students on the ISU campus. My two fellow nursing students and I shared a bedroom. One Mennonite roommate had a car, so the other two of us chipped in for gas as transportation to Mennonite for class and clinicals. If she was unavailable, then a taxi, bus, or walking was the mode of transportation. The nice apartment was located in a safe area and had one bathroom, a kitchen, a dining area, a living area, plus two bedrooms.

Our new living arrangement worked well, but not without challenges. One of my ISU friends decided to get married and did not return to school, leaving a vacant spot. For the first part of the semester, this spot was filled by a wonderful girl who was a good fit, and we all got along fine. However, she was only committed for part of the semester. The remainder of the semester, we experienced the hippie lifestyle firsthand. Our new roommate and her friends were more of the "free spirit" persuasion. As nursing students, we had early morning clinicals necessitating leaving the apartment by 6:30 am to arrive at the hospital by 7 am. Several mornings, we woke up to strangers sleeping on our living room floor. I'm reasonably certain marijuana was in our midst from time to time as well. Thankfully, we established some expectations preventing things from getting totally out of control.

Because we were responsible for our meals, we three nurses pooled our culinary knowledge and avoided starvation. We grocery-shopped together and planned our menu for the week. As I recall, lunch would have been eaten at the hospital, we had our separate breakfast preferences, and dinner was eaten together. One of our favorite meals was hot tuna sandwiches made with tuna, egg, mayo, and cheese, plopped in a hot dog bun, wrapped in foil, and baked until it was warm. We also made pork chops. I am certain my fabulous cheese sauce would have been slathered on something from time to time.

That semester was not without some unsettling moments. On one occasion, one of the girls from the apartment below us became angry with us for reasons I do not recall. When I opened the door in response to her knocking, she stood wielding a large knife and loudly threatening me. Being from a small town, I had never experienced anything like this. Another time, I decided to walk the eight blocks to ISU after dark to visit Kay Beth. It was common for women to be out walking on the campus in the evening, and although I was somewhat concerned, I went anyway. As I was nearing her dorm, I heard someone running behind me. I stepped to the side of the sidewalk to allow the person to pass, but when he got up to me, instead of passing me as I had anticipated, he grabbed me. When I screamed, fortunately he ran away without harming me. Instead of visiting my friend, I spent the evening at the police station reporting the incident, which found its way into the newspaper. I do not recommend this as a way of gaining notoriety.

Our apartment contract covered only the first semester, forcing us to find living arrangements for the second semester. My roommate was familiar with the Bloomington area and knew a man with an apartment in a house we could rent. I reconnected with a summer school friend, so the four of us–three Mennonite girls and one ISU student–rented the apartment. Although a serviceable place, it was certainly no frills. Located on the third floor of a large home, most likely a renovated attic, we had two bedrooms, one bathroom, a living room, and a small kitchen. The apartment was accessed through an outdoor wooden staircase with a small landing at the top. Everything was carried up three flights of outside stairs – groceries, suitcases, laundry, books, everything. The windows were little more than dormer windows with pigeons roosting right outside. I recall waking up to the sound of pigeons cooing and looking out the small windows to see them roosting directly outside. Knocking on the windows encouraged them to vacate their roosting place.

As if that was not enough, our landlord was apparently engaged in a property line dispute with the next-door neighbor. While we were living there, the neighbor erected a wooden fence on the property line located about a foot from the stairway. We could barely fit through the narrow space with groceries, suitcases, books, and anything we had to carry. I recall walking sideways to get through to access the stairway. The apartment was within easy walking distance of Mennonite Hospital. When working at the switchboard, I could walk to work and take a cab home after dark.

Senior year clinical time increased to 16 – 24 hours per week. Our clinical experience included one week of the evening shift and one week on the night shift. We learned increasingly complex skills as we honed our nursing judgment, addressed increasingly complex situations, started IVs, and administered IV medications.

## IV Administration

As seniors, the complexity of our skills and breadth of knowledge continued expanding. All aspects of intravenous (IV) administration were learned from inserting the needle into the vein and infusing fluids into the body to IV medication administration. Accessing a vein and starting the IV was learned by starting IVs on each other. IVs are inserted by locating the vein via sight, i.e. "visualizing" the vein and feeling it. Veins are distended by applying a tourniquet to the upper arm to block the flow of blood returning to the heart, making them easier to palpate and spot. We used butterfly needles rather than the plastic catheters that are used today. The butterfly needles had two "wings" which folded onto each other leaving the needle free. When the vein was located, we held the needle parallel to the vein and inserted it at a slight angle. We were taught to bring the point of the needle right to the vein and then puncture the vein's wall with the needle. We knew we had "hit" the vein or entered the vein because we could feel a "pop" as the needle punctured the venous wall. Although the antecubital space in the crook of the arm is the largest and most easily accessible vein, we usually chose a vein in the hand or wrist to allow the patient to use his/her arm. Butterfly needles were smaller gauge and rigid, predisposing them to blockage by blood clots. Because these rigid needles lacked flexibility, they could potentially penetrate the vein over time, leading to infiltration of the IV, making them inferior to today's plastic IV catheters.

Pumps that automatically calculate the amount of fluid infusing into the patient were unavailable, and IV bottles were glass rather than the current plastic bags. Regular IV tubing is 10 – 20 drops per milliliter of fluid. Micro-drip tubing is 60 drops per milliliter of fluid. Nurses calculated the rate by holding their watch up to the drip chamber and calculating the number of drops per minute using the watch's second hand. At the same time, the nurse manipulated the roller clamp on the IV tubing to achieve the prescribed rate of the drip.

If a medication was added to the IV, the nurse calculated the number of drops per minute to achieve the dose, usually without assistance from the Pharmacist. To avoid a disastrous patient safety event, medication bottle labels were carefully scrutinized to make sure the medication was intended for IV use. The IV bottle was labeled with the medication, dose, and infusion time. It was possible for the nurse to carefully establish an accurate drip rate, only to check on the IV at an acceptable interval and find the bottle empty or not infusing at all. Patient arm movement and position might alter the drip rate, or a clot might form at the needle point requiring it to be irrigated or changed.

Micro drip chambers were challenging because the micro drip tubing contained regular IV tubing plus a reservoir attached to the IV bottle. The trick was to maintain an accurate flow of drips from the micro drip chamber by making sure the chamber always contained fluid. Regular IV tubing was used for adults, but the micro drip chamber might be used to administer medications. The micro drip system was also commonly used to administer fluids and medication to infants and children. Because the fluid would not infuse into the patient unless the chamber was full, it was frustrating to constantly make sure that the chamber contained fluid. Using the second hand of our watch, we calculated the drip by counting 60 drops per minute to achieve the desired dose. Maintaining that dose was often a moving target. Today's IV pumps were a welcome addition to the medical equipment armamentarium.

**Psychiatric Nursing**

In the spirit of transparency, I can disclose that although I found the psychiatric rotation interesting, psychiatric nursing was my least favorite rotation. Having revealed that, I admit that when I returned to graduate school, my favorite class of all time was Psychopathology, the study of mental, emotional, and behavioral disorders. I found the study of various mental health illnesses and diagnoses fascinating. However, I have never felt called to work with mentally ill patients. My interest in the clinical picture does not translate to a desire to care for patients who are mentally ill. I admire the dedicated nurses working in that specialty because it is definitely a calling requiring a special person.

The Psychiatric rotation consisted of two components. The first part of the rotation was spent on the Psychiatric ward at Brokaw Hospital in Normal, Illinois. The second part of the rotation was spent commuting to Peoria State Hospital in Bartonville, Illinois. (My mother sometimes said I was going to drive her to Bartonville, meaning I needed to stop being so difficult because I was unduly taxing her child-rearing coping mechanisms. My husband's mother always said her children's behavior would drive her to Elgin – same concept, different location.) As in other rotations, we were assigned six or eight students to a group and rotated our time with other groups.

The experience at Brokaw Hospital differed from Peoria State Hospital in that the hospitalized Brokaw patients had a high level of functionality. They might have been hospitalized for an exacerbation of symptoms, alcoholism, newly diagnosed mental health issues, or observation regarding a change in their mental status. Electroshock therapy was a common treatment and was administered much like it is today. I recall giving oral paraldehyde to an alcoholic patient to relax him as he endured the stages of alcohol withdrawal. It smelled as bad as it sounds, and I felt sorry for anyone having to drink it.

I found this rotation challenging because the patient's symptoms were often subtle. To establish equilibrium, the students had to reconcile the purpose of hospitalizing these patients when the patient might appear "normal". As we interacted with the seasoned mental health staff, we learned that establishing equilibrium is a rite of passage when working with the mentally ill. The patient's mental illness is not always readily identified, and the patient can present as psychologically intact. However, as we probed beyond the patient's superficial behavior, the mental health issues became apparent and were recognized. Having never been exposed to these behavioral issues, it was a very unique world that required some adjustment on the student's part.

Peoria State Hospital was a different story. Based on their symptoms, these patients left no doubt regarding their mental illness. As with the Pediatric rotation, we were the first class not required to LIVE on the hospital grounds for four weeks. When I saw the living accommodations, I was very thankful we were allowed to commute from

Bloomington to Bartonville and return to our apartment after our clinical day. The state hospital dorm rooms were dark, drab, and dingy, with single metal beds. Although the grounds were pretty, the property was isolated from stores, entertainment, and civilization. Our group of student nurses was relieved to bypass this residential experience.

Peoria State Hospital was founded as the Illinois Asylum for the Incurably Insane in 1895. Construction in Bartonville, Illinois, was completed in 1897, and the facility received its first patients in 1902. Its purpose was to house mentally ill patients diagnosed as incurable. Patients were referred to Bartonville from facilities throughout the state. The hospital participated in a psychiatric nursing affiliation program for nursing students from 1943 to 1969. At its peak in the 1950s, the hospital housed 2,800 patients. After its closure was announced in 1972, the patient census dropped to 600. It is registered by the National Park Service as a historic site and was featured on the TV show *Ghost Hunters* (Peoria State Hospital, 2023).

With 215 acres and 63 buildings, it made quite an impression on our group of young nursing students. After touring the campus, our student group selected the men's maximum-security ward as the patient population for our clinical experience. I do not recall why we chose that particular patient population, but I do recall that once we arrived on our assigned day and entered the building, the door was locked behind us, leaving us locked in with the patients. I never felt fearful in that environment because the patients were controlled with ample staff to watch over us. However, I did consider the significance of being locked in a ward comprised entirely of mentally ill men. One day as our student nurse group entered, we heard a significant commotion in the intake room. The male supervisor instructed the nursing students to avoid proximity to that room because a violent patient was being restrained and immobilized to the bed. It must have required significant manpower to subdue the patient because the room was full of people. The student nurses complied, and none of us went near the room.

The male patients were housed in a two-story structure with the activity and living spaces on the first floor and the large, open sleeping area located on the second floor. The entire sleeping area held row after row of stark metal patient beds covered with white sheets, blankets, and pillows. The open sleeping arrangement provided no privacy for the patients. I'm unsure where or how the patients stored their minimal personal belongings. Each student was paired with one patient from the ward, with a majority of the clinical rotation spent interacting with that patient. Each student nurse studied her patient's psychiatric disease(s), including symptoms, treatment, and prognosis. The student then observed and assessed her patient while monitoring the patient's behavior and response to the treatment regimen. The student nurse compiled an individualized care plan to enhance the patient's quality of life and prognosis.

My patient was a middle-aged man diagnosed with schizophrenia. Schizophrenia is a mental health disorder that interferes with a person's ability to think, feel, or behave clearly. A person diagnosed with schizophrenia may have thoughts or emotions that appear out of touch with reality. Their speech and behavior are often disorganized, they experience difficulty participating in daily activities, and they most likely have altered concentration.

My patient had a history of running away from the facility, and upon arriving one Monday morning, I was informed that he had run away that weekend. I spent many hours with him as I interviewed him, assessed his illness, and got to know him. We spent time in the unit, in conference rooms, walking the grounds (when he was allowed outside), and participating in group meetings. One of my classmates had been paired with him for the previous rotation, and she said he ran away as the end of her clinical rotation drew near. The patient exhibited the same behavior when my clinical rotation ended. As my departure drew near, he ran away. I felt sorry for these patients who developed a relationship with the student assigned to them for a few weeks, only to have that student vanish from their lives.

In addition to the one-on-one time with our patients, we attended group therapy sessions and some classes. It was an interesting time. Little did I know that my very last career work assignment would be providing consulting services at three mental health facilities. And that is also a story for a different day.

For the students' last day on campus, we hosted a party for the patients. We furnished treats, and the hospital provided a bowl of punch. I recall that one of the patients dropped his lit cigarette in the punch shortly after the party began. And that, as they say, was that.

### Emergency Room

Our Emergency Room (ER) rotation (referred to as the Emergency Room back then and the Emergency Department now) was only a few weeks long. Mennonite's small ER department consisted of one major room and two minor rooms. Due to the size and limited resources available in Mennonite's ER, patients experiencing a serious illness or injury were likely to be transferred to a hospital equipped to handle a higher patient acuity level.

Since central Illinois is home to vast farmland, farm injuries were always potential emergencies. Farm equipment is hazardous and unforgiving, capable of inflicting critical and life-threatening injuries to soft tissue, organs, and bones. Sometimes the extensive damage leads to shock, and if not treated quickly, the patient dies. Dirt, manure, or chemicals may complicate the injury, resulting in complex trauma inflicted on the human body. Although the patient might survive the initial trauma, he/she could later succumb to infection. During one of my shifts, a patient who had sustained a significant traumatic farm equipment injury was brought in. He was the most critically injured patient that I had witnessed up to that time. Because of his extensive life-threatening injuries, he was transferred by ambulance to the higher level of care offered at St. Francis Hospital in Peoria, Illinois. While performing a thorough assessment of his injuries, IVs were started. He was prepared for ambulance transport, and the receiving hospital was notified. My fellow nursing student and I were allowed to accompany the patient in the ambulance for his transfer to St. Francis Hospital in Peoria, Illinois. We were seated in the back of the ambulance with the patient, the paramedics, and another RN from Mennonite as we sped to Peoria with flashing lights and sirens. Upon arrival, my fellow nursing student and I accompanied the patient and our team into the ER at St. Francis to observe the patient's treatment in their large, bustling department. Once the patient was settled and the handoff report was given to their team, the ambulance returned us to Bloomington. We two student nurses undoubtedly had clinicals the next day, making it a short but exciting night.

## Team Leading

The nursing professional practice model establishes how nurses will practice at their organization to achieve the best clinical outcome for the patient. The care delivery model flows from the professional practice model and outlines how care will be provided. The care delivery model for most organizations was team nursing. As mentioned previously, team nursing came about due to the lack of available nurses to perform total patient care. Each care delivery team consisted of ancillary staff, including nursing assistants and licensed practical nurses working under the direction of a single RN.

Each student nurse attended the change of shift report as the oncoming nursing team leader. The outgoing RN provided a summary of each patient, including his/her name, age, physician(s), diagnosis, treatments, IV fluids, infusion rate, medications, patient response to their illness, activity level, tests, and pertinent demographic and social information. As students, we learned the plan for each of our patients that day, and the number of surgeries and anticipated discharges for our team. Before leaving the change of shift report, the team leader communicated patient assignments to each team member and discussed patient goals for the shift.

Hospitalists, physicians hired by the hospital to assume 24-hour care for inpatients, were not part of the healthcare system then. Each patient's personal doctor assumed total responsibility for his/her hospitalized patients' care. The physicians usually arrived at the hospital early to complete morning rounds before office hours started. As the team leader, the student nurse accompanied the physicians as they visited and examined each of their patients. During the rounds, the student communicated the patient's progress and current status to the physician. Being present during the physician's examination allowed the student nurse to hear the physician's opinion and orders in real-time. Learning the physician's findings firsthand provided accurate information to communicate to our team and the next team during the change-of-shift report. Revisions to the treatment plan were communicated before entering it into the chart. The physician often returned to the hospital in the evening to check on their patients. Lack of 24-hour on-site physician coverage meant that the patient's physician was contacted for any issues or status changes affecting their patients.

The ancillary staff completed basic patient care and some treatments, while we students passed medications and completed more complex patient care. Nearly EVERYTHING was handwritten. Physician orders transcribed by the Unit Clerk were reviewed for accuracy and signed off by the RN before being added to the Kardex by the Unit Clerk. We notified the physician of any questions. New medications were ordered through the hospital pharmacy and distributed to the unit.

As the team leader, the student nurses led team conferences where the entire team assembled for 15-20 minutes to conduct an in-depth review of a patient from the unit. The team reviewed the plan of care and evaluated achievement of the goals outlined in that plan. Subsequent nursing interventions were revised and implemented based on the evaluation to meet the treatment goals and outcomes. Any revisions to the existing plan were documented by hand in the patient's Kardex. The student nurse's team leader rotation provided a realistic experience for our future role as a floor nurse. Experiencing team leader responsibilities as a student built the necessary skills to lead the nursing team, communicate with the ancillary staff, and coordinate the care of numerous patients with the healthcare team.

As senior student nurses, we learned to cultivate professionalism – not only in how we presented ourselves, but also in how we perceived our roles and identities as future nurses. We had matured and moved beyond the 18-year-old novice students of three years prior. We were transitioning into professional nurses with a meaningful career ahead of us. We carried ourselves with more confidence. We were senior nursing students with the black band across our nursing caps to prove it. Underclassmen looked up to us. We started formulating post-graduation plans and began preparing to physically and emotionally leave the safety of our school for the real world of healthcare.

Senior nursing students were allowed to elect an additional two-week rotation in the specialty of their choice. Of course, I chose to spend two extra weeks in surgery. The staff welcomed me into the OR world and allowed me to build on the skills learned in my junior year. I was given additional opportunities to scrub, circulate, and prepare the room. Because the staff knew me, they encouraged me to participate in the surgical cases. It was an enjoyable two weeks because feeling more confident and comfortable in the environment allowed me to relax and engage with the procedures and the people, sealing my desire to work in the OR. I was sad to leave when the two weeks ended.

**The Autopsy and the Cadaver**

As death is part of the life cycle, so it was also understandably part of our nursing education. In addition to caring for people who died in the hospital, I had an opportunity to observe people who were already dead by witnessing an autopsy and working on a cadaver.

One afternoon, our nursing class was invited by a local funeral home to observe an autopsy if we wished to attend. We did not have long to decide because the autopsy was scheduled in a couple of hours. Those in our class who elected to go accompanied the instructor the couple of blocks to the funeral home. When our student group arrived in the autopsy room, the body of an elderly woman was lying naked on a white marble table. To be very blunt, an autopsy provides the opportunity to more clearly visualize organs without the hindrance of blood and body fluids obstructing the view. Although not an experience I wish to replicate, I'm glad I went.

The autopsy began when the physician made a long incision down the middle of the patient's body. He then removed the heart, lungs, liver, stomach, kidneys, pancreas, and other structures. As the physician removed each organ, he explained the anatomy of that organ, pointing out the various sections or parts. Each organ was weighed, and the disease process was identified and documented. At the autopsy conclusion, the physician closed the skin of the massive incision using a large suture. There was no need for a cosmetic closure; just put the body back together.

A friend of Terry's was enrolled in a Human Anatomy class and invited me to join him as he worked on the cadaver he was dissecting. After some hesitation, I decided to accompany him to the human anatomy lab at ISU. The cadavers were housed in large individual vats containing some type of fluid (probably formaldehyde) for preservation. The cadaver was accessed by a foot pedal that lifted the cadaver out of the vat when compressed. Fortunately, Mr. Cadaver's head was contained in plastic, preventing me from seeing his face. Terry's friend was working on the legs and groin. We could clearly discern the nerves, veins, arteries, and muscles. I concentrated on the area where he was working because taking in the entire body made the experience difficult. Cadavers aren't pretty. Although our nursing education provided two semesters of Anatomy and Physiology, we were not required to take Human Anatomy. I was grateful for the opportunity to spend an afternoon with a cadaver, but glad I wasn't required to do it again.

## Memorable Patients

Obtaining a nursing education is a life-altering endeavor that has touched me mentally and emotionally. Three patients made an indelible impression on me. One, of course, was my Obstetrics patient whom I referenced earlier. Two more provide vivid memories of the experience of caring for them.

The first was a woman in her mid-40s suffering from the final stages of metastatic colon cancer. Hospice was first introduced in 1974, so in 1969, patients nearing the end of life often died in the hospital. I cared for this patient on a Sunday evening shift while working as a Nursing Assistant at the hospital. Working as a Nursing Assistant generated income and provided a great opportunity to develop clinical skills. I was assigned to this patient and four or five other patients. I recall that she was emaciated, pale, and very weak. Although chemotherapy existed, it was not as sophisticated as it is today. Lack of effective cancer drugs or complex chemotherapy resulted in cancer often being a death sentence. Her situation evoked feelings of sorrow and compassion. I was emotionally touched by her because of her age and because she had young children at home. It was obvious that she was dying with little time left. After taking her vital signs and providing as much comfort as possible, I learned that she had a fecal impaction, most likely resulting from the pain medication and inactivity. The fecal impaction had to be removed, and I was the one who had to remove it. This is distasteful for the one removing it and very uncomfortable/painful for the patient. Rather than feeling repulsed, I felt compassion for this patient and her plight. I dutifully got the blue protective pad, gloves, and lubricant and set to task. As the patient lay on her side, I entered her rectum and literally "dug out" the hard clumps of fecal matter and placed them on the blue pad. It was a laborious process due to her fragile condition and the discomfort caused by the procedure. I was seldom bothered by the smell or sight of bodily functions. I think I focused on the job at hand rather than focusing on how disgusting everything looked. Anyway, I got her "cleaned out". Following the manual extraction, she most likely received an enema to finish the fecal evacuation. We were both grateful when the exhausting ordeal was done.

I vividly recall the day she died a week or so later. I was working at the switchboard as the gurney carrying her black body bag was wheeled past the switchboard to the waiting hearse. As a young woman of 20, I sat at the switchboard and contemplated what this woman's death meant, how her life was over, and the impending impact on her family. I was struck with the realization that she must have died alone because I do not recall any family members accompanying the body.

The second patient was a prominent member of the community, newly diagnosed with a malignant brain tumor. Her room was adorned with beautiful flower arrangements from friends and professional colleagues. When I entered her room to meet her, she was beautifully dressed in her nightgown and matching chiffon bed jacket. Although shocked by the diagnosis, she attempted to maintain a positive attitude. Her many visitors wished her well and provided emotional support. This was my first experience caring for someone considered a VIP. I was initially intimidated by the entire situation and caring for someone so well-known in the community. However, as I spent time with her, the intimidation faded as I got to know her and cared for her.

The small wooden plaque she kept on her bedside table caught my attention. It quoted Matthew 6:33 and read, "Do not worry about tomorrow, for tomorrow will worry about its own things. Sufficient for the day is its own trouble". As a new Christian, this plaque spoke to me and I was to refer to Matthew 6:33 often in the days and months ahead. She was to have many more admissions to the hospital. I recall that she sought a second opinion at a larger medical center, but returned to our hospital numerous times before she finally succumbed to the disease.

**Marriage**

*A cord of three strands is not quickly broken. Ecclesiastes 4:12*

And sometimes life happens. I never imagined getting married while still in school, but having a boyfriend in the military provided a dimension of unpredictability. Add to that the fact that our country was at war in Vietnam, and war influences and impacts situations with more disorganization than peacetime. Weddings weren't planned for a "year from now" or "two years from now" because, with someone in the military, there was no way to predict how life would look in one year, two years, or even six months.

Following basic training, Terry was selected for Cryptanalyst training and transferred to Fort Devens, Massachusetts, where he was stationed for about a year. The physical distance between us had widened, and the time spent together had narrowed. He was much farther away than Fort Leonard Wood, Missouri, and our time spent together was reduced to holidays.

One evening in mid-February 1971, Terry called and asked me to marry him, stating that he was scheduled for leave in nine weeks. After accepting his proposal, I was now on a fast track to a wedding in a little over two months. That timeline would soon be accelerated. He called back two nights later and said his leave was moved up to six weeks from now, and could we get married in six weeks? The fast track now became lightning-fast. It was the middle of February, and our wedding date was set for April 3, 1971.

Everything began moving in high gear just a few days after we became engaged. The following Saturday, his mother and my two future sisters-in-law met my parents and me at Bergner's Department Store in Peoria, Illinois to choose my wedding gown, veil, and bridesmaid dresses. With six weeks of lead time, my wedding gown selection quickly narrowed down to those dresses that would arrive in time. I recall trying on an ivory lace dress, and the group said, "No, that looks like a tablecloth". Not wishing to be married in a tablecloth, we progressed to the remaining dresses. I had dreamed of a dress with a long train, but the dress I chose had a relatively short train. My future sister-in-law, an excellent seamstress, agreed to attach a longer veil to the headpiece I selected. I had my long train after all.

I was thankful to have my future sisters-in-law with me to select the bridesmaid dresses. I loved our choice of beautiful long-sleeved floor-length pink chiffon dresses with white lace trim. I think everyone liked them, at least I hoped they did. We picked out the headdresses to match. Except for my sisters-in-law, my attendants didn't see their dresses until the day before the wedding, when the necessary alterations were made. Fortunately, only minor alterations were required.

After bidding my future family goodbye for their return trip to Rockford, I sat for my engagement picture. My parents and I then traveled to Morton, Illinois, where we selected the cake, flowers, and invitations. Although I wasn't overly picky about the cake and the flowers, I had seen pictures of bridesmaid bouquets that I liked. They were round, covered in small mums, and carried by a pink ribbon. I thought they were beautiful, and the florist agreed to make them.

Central Illinois wedding receptions were simple in 1971 and usually held in the church parlor, i.e. basement, eliminating the need to reserve a reception venue and engage a caterer. At traditional receptions, cake, sometimes ice cream, nuts, mints, and punch were served. Because our wedding included out-of-town guests, my mother arranged a simple buffet lunch for our reception.

Weekends were filled with preparation and planning activities. We met with the photographer, had my wedding photograph taken in my gown and veil, addressed and mailed invitations, completed the bridal registry, purchased Terry's wedding ring, and planned any outstanding details. Terry was not present for any of this planning, but he seemed pleased with the outcome of everything.

Bridal showers were held in Rockford and my hometown over the next few weekends. My fellow nursing students hosted a shower at the dorm. My parents' basement resembled the appliance department at Macy's.

In the meantime, Terry traveled to New York City to purchase my engagement and wedding rings from his friend's uncle's jewelry store. During his short trip, he enjoyed some of New York City's attractions. I was the lucky recipient of his sparkling purchase.

Terry arrived home the week before our wedding and slipped the beautiful engagement ring on my finger. After driving from Rockford, he arrived at my apartment with our shiny new 1971 light blue Volkswagen Beetle. I am grateful he taught me how to drive a stick shift on our first date because I would be left to maneuver the car up and down the hills of Bloomington.

Throughout this wedding planning frenzy, I remained a senior in nursing school, which required all my time and attention. I attended classes and clinicals until the day or two before my wedding. I recall that I was excused from classes on Friday to be married on Saturday.

April 3$^{rd}$ was a beautiful, sunny day in Manito, perfect for a spring wedding. Because out-of-town guests were in the wedding party and I had a tight school schedule, the rehearsal was held Saturday morning, the day of the wedding, followed by the rehearsal lunch. After lunch, everyone converged on my parents' home for last-minute preparations. I remember my former roommate and I sitting at my parents' kitchen table crying, both of us. I am unsure what prompted both of us to cry, but cry we did.

We proceeded to the church where I applied my makeup and my cousin styled my hair. I watched from the dressing room window as my husband-to-be was carried up the church stairs by his groomsmen. I still love that picture.

The wedding flew by, and I transitioned from Miss Ila Ethell to Mrs. Ila Minnick. There would be no honeymoon because I was still in school and Terry was in the Army. And there was a war on, a very terrible war. I am thankful we didn't know how that war would impact our lives in the coming months. We spent our wedding night at the Holiday Inn in Pekin, Illinois. I was to tell my husband goodbye a few days after our wedding and return to school for my clinicals. Knowing that I would not see my new husband for two months made for a difficult goodbye.

# 7

## Graduation and Moving On

*There is a time for everything and a season for every activity under the heavens. Ecclesiastes 3:1*

Three years flew by. I had gained a new name, and a brand-new career lay ahead of me. My classmates and I were euphoric as difficult final exams were written and the last clinicals attended. There was a tradition that on the next-to-last day of school, the graduating nurses cut each other's student nurse uniforms with their bandage scissors. Sometimes there was an element of surprise as we snuck up on our unsuspecting classmate and snip, snipped their uniform. By the end of that day, most of us were wearing rags as we let off steam and engaged in uproarious laughter. Preparing for our upcoming goodbyes made for a bittersweet day.

To celebrate the conclusion of our education, we wore white nursing uniforms on our last day of clinicals. We were so proud to have completed our education as we walked to our final clinical assignment dressed as professional nurses. Our student uniforms would henceforth be memorabilia from our nursing school days. The photo section contains a picture of my junior-year roommate and me standing in front of the nursing dorm.

Three years prior, we had entered school as mostly 18-year-olds fresh out of high school. We were strangers who became cherished friends. We laughed together, cried together, and experienced student life together. Members of our class broke up with high school sweethearts, married high school sweethearts, met our future husbands, and in some cases married our future husbands, had babies, shared our past lives, moved on from our childhood, and pursued our future dreams. We transitioned from timid novice student nurses to blossoming professional women ready to assume our place in healthcare.

All too quickly, it was time to leave Mennonite. On June 21, 1971, a beautiful Sunday in June, we proudly donned our freshly pressed white graduation uniforms, crisp white hose, spotless white shoes, and nursing caps as we stepped forward to receive our diplomas and school pins. My parents, grandparents, and a few college friends were in attendance. I was elated as I walked down the long aisle at Wesley United Methodist Church to that magnificent pipe organ processing us in. To celebrate our graduation, the choir sang, an inspirational speaker shared their message, and Dr. Kinder addressed the audience. Before we knew it, the ceremony had ended, and we were officially graduates. Following graduation, the school provided a lovely reception in our honor at the church.

And then it was time to say goodbye. We hugged one another with promises to get together. However, those promises wouldn't materialize for another 15 years when we had our first reunion. Saying goodbye to my former roommate was emotional for both of us. After that day, I only saw her one other time for the rest of my life. I never saw some of my friends in that graduating class again. Although we had several reunions, not every classmate attended.

The day before graduation, my parents and I packed the 1971 blue Volkswagen with all of my earthly belongings for my move to Massachusetts to join my husband. We crammed that car with our dishes, pots and pans, sheets, bath towels, kitchen towels, an iron, an ironing board, some kitchen utensils, my clothes, and my parents' luggage.

Following graduation, the reception, and a few graduation pictures, we were off! I departed my graduation in my nursing uniform, excluding the cap, and my parents and I headed East. We had space for two people in the front and just enough room in the backseat for one person. Every other square inch was filled with household items, clothing, and more than likely some snacks. We drove as far as Richmond, Indiana that first night. In two days, we entered Fort Devens, Massachusetts, where my husband met us. Now there were three people in the front seat and one person in the back seat of that little car, but we were happy to finally be together.

Terry had rented a modest little apartment for us. Our kind landlords allowed us to pay weekly rent, so no lease was required. Because we would only be in Massachusetts for three months, I did not pursue employment. Our apartment was in a spacious, older home that had been converted into multiple units. Moving in required little labor and minimal time because one little blue Volkswagen contained our entire household. Being a "furnished" apartment translated to Terry and me rummaging through the attic and scrounging around until we found "suitable" furniture. We scavenged a bed and dresser, two "living room" chairs, and a drop-leaf kitchen table with two chairs. That was it. I adorned a cardboard box with contact paper to serve as an end table between the chairs. We had no TV unless our neighbor loaned us hers if she was away. We purchased a "stereo" consisting of a radio, turntable, and cassette tape player and checked out "records" from the local library.

Our summer was filled with adventure, residing in a new area rich with history and beautiful scenery. I spent my days reading, caring for our little apartment, learning to cook, and simply being a new wife. We enjoyed the tourist activities that our military salary would allow. Many weekends were spent strolling around Boston, going to the beach, including Cape Cod, or driving around the countryside. Our food budget was $10 a week, and we saved our change to dine out.

With Cryptanalyst school nearing completion, Terry was scheduled to receive his next orders around the first part of August. We excitedly anticipated his next assignment, thinking we might be sent to Germany or even stateside. The possibility of his being sent to Vietnam never entered our minds. Previous Cryptanalyst classes had been sent to Europe, and some even remained stateside, leading us to wrongly conclude that our experience would be the same. I sent him off to the base that morning with no worry or dread of what might be coming next. When he arrived home, he was sullen. I excitedly inquired, "Where are we going"? When he uttered the word "Vietnam," I was in shock. He had already stopped at the home of friends to settle himself before he came and told me. I just sank into our kitchen chair in disbelief. Terry sat across the table from me. There would be no exciting assignment in Europe, no stateside residence. There would only be a year-long separation a few months into this marriage. We resigned ourselves to what would ultimately happen and began making plans. It was decided that I would live in Rockford. Terry wanted me to live with his mother. I would get a job at one of the local hospitals, hopefully in the operating room, and with God's help and protection, we would endure this separation.

We left Massachusetts on Labor Day weekend, 1971, and drove back to Illinois. It was a long, hot drive in a car with no air conditioning. Before his departure, we traveled back and forth between Rockford and Manito, staying with my parents and his mother. Terry left for Vietnam on September 30, 1971.

# Epilogue

*The Lord is close to the brokenhearted and saves the crushed in spirit. Psalm 34:18*

By the time Terry left for Vietnam, I had moved my clothing and personal items into the little bedroom I was to occupy at Terry's mother's home. Our household items – dishes, pots and pans, linens- were stored at my parents' home because we had no home to set up.

I vividly remember the day he left. It was September 30, 1971, a sunny fall day, and one day after Terry's 23rd birthday. His canvas sack was dutifully packed with uniforms, boots, and personal items, all tucked inside. As we prepared for the day, we felt empty, spent, and sick. The goodbyes began early with his mother first. We had lunch at his sister's house with her family, Terry's father, and Terry's best friend who would drive him to the airport. It was a gut-wrenching nightmare, like watching ominous storm clouds gather, powerless to stop the impending tempest. With great sorrow, we faced the realization of no guarantees of ever seeing one another again – literally. How does one possibly say goodbye in those circumstances? Terry was crying, I was crying. It is just an impossible feeling, knowing that this is happening and nothing can be done about it. We hugged one another, kissed each other goodbye, promised to write every day, and to pray for one another. And with that, he was out the door, in the car, and backing out of the driveway. I watched his friend's red Ford Galaxy from the back door until he was out of sight.

I would begin my first job as a Graduate Nurse four days later. Because my state board licensing exams were scheduled for the same day Terry left for Vietnam, I postponed taking them. The next available testing dates were January 1972, forcing me to wait longer than planned to write my state boards. As a result of this decision, I had to work as a Graduate Nurse (GN) rather than a Registered Nurse (RN). Thankfully, my supervisor was understanding, and the department accommodated the necessary delay in my status.

My professional nursing journey began on October 4, 1971, when I started my first job in the operating room at Rockford Memorial Hospital, Rockford, Illinois. I was to spend over 50 years working, with most of that time spent in or around the operating room. But that, as they say, is a story for another day and will be captured in my next book, *"Keeping You in Stitches"*.

# References

About nursing diploma programs (2012). https://nursingexplorer.com/diploma#googlevignette.

Ang, R. (2019). *Nursing kardex: Patient care summary. Canadian Journal of Informatics Vol 14(3)*. https://cjni.net/?p=6338.

Association, American Nurses (2021). *Nursing scope and standards of practice. American Nurses Association.* ISBN 978-0-9993088-6-8. https://en.m.wikipedia.org/wiki/Nursing (2025, January 21).

Berg, C. (1865). Day by day and with each passing moment. In Hymns for the Family of God (1976). Word Music.

Cipriano, P. (2010). *The world of nursing – then and now. American Nurse.* https://www.myamericannurse.com/the-world-of-nursing-then-and-now.

College of Nursing, Mennonite (1985). *The passing of the flame, Mennonite College of Nursing History Books* (Book 2). http://ir.library.illinoisstate.edu/mcnflame/2.

*Florence Nightingale pledge.* (2010). https://nursing.vanderbilt.edu/news/florence-nightingale-pledge/.

Garet, L. (2020). *History of MRIs and the evolution of this life-saving technology.* https://ezra.com/blog/history-of-mri-scans.

Hallett, C. (2010). *Celebrating nurses: A visual history.* Hauppauge, NY: Barron's Educational Services, Inc.

Hehman, M., Keeling, A., & Kirchgessner, J. (2018). History of professional nursing in the United States. New York, NY: Springer Publishing Co.

Hoover, N.L. and T.F. Kapp, (1985). Mennonite Hospital School of Nursing: The passing of the flame. Bloomington, Illinois, USA: Global Anabaptist Mennonite Encyclopedia Online. Retrieved 21 February 2024, https://gameo.org/index.php?title=Mennonite_Hospital_School_of_Nursing_(Bloomington,_,_USA)&oldid=90751.

Hoover, N. O. and T. F. Kaap. (1957). Mennonite Hospital School of Nursing (Bloomington, Illinois, USA). Global Anabaptist Mennonite Encyclopedia Online. https://gameo.org/index.php?title=Mennonite_Hospital_School_of_Nursing_(Bloomington,_Illinois,_USA)&oldid=89751.

Kumar, D. (2023). Basic principles and history of CT scan, pptx. https://www.slideshare.net/dheerajkumar838/basic-principles-and-history-of-ct-scanpptx.

Mennonite College of Nursing (2024). BSN plan of study. https://Plan of Study | Mennonite College of Nursing - Illinois State.

Mennonite Hospital School of Nursing (1970). School of Nursing Catalog.
Mount-Campbell AF, Evans KD, Woods DD, Chipps E, Moffatt-Bruce SD, Patel K, Patterson ES, (2020). Uncovering the value of a historical paper-based collaborative artifact: The nursing unit's kardex system. Front Digit Health. 2020 Aug 7;2:12. doi: 10.3389/fdgth.2020.00012. PMID: 34713025; PMCID: PMC8521873.
https://www.ncbi.nlm.nih.gov/pmc/articles/PMC8521873/.

Nurse Groups (2018). The story of Florence Nightingale, https://www.nursegroups.com/nursing-article/the-story-of-florence-nightingale.html.

Nurse Journal, (March, 2023), https://nursejournal.org/articles/the-number-of-male-nurses-has-multiplied-10x-in-the-past-40-years/.
*Pharmacology*, Wikipedia Foundation, (2024, November 17). https://en.wikipedia.org/wiki/Pharmacology.

Schutt, B. (1961). in Hehman, M., Keeling, A., & Kirchgessner, J. (2018). *History of professional nursing in the United States*. New York, NY: Springer Publishing Co.

Selanders, L. & Crane, P. (2010). Florence Nightingale in absentia: nursing and the 1893 Columbian Exposition. Journal of Holistic Nursing, Dec;28(4):305-312. Doi:10.1177/0898010110361523. Epub2010 Aug 31. PMID: 20807865.

Singleton, M. (2020). Flashback Friday - *Practice makes perfect: The history of simulation*, Excerpted from "Where Role Play Meets Reality," by Sarah Craig, PhD, RN, CCNS, CCRN-K, CHSE, and Bethany Cieslowski, DNP, MA, RN, CHSE, presented at the 2019 American Association for the History of Nursing conference. Retrieved from History of Simulation • UVA School of Nursing (virginia.edu).

University Staff. (2023-2024 issue). *New Mennonite College of Nursing simulation lab opens. The Flame*. Mennonite College of Nursing at Illinois State University.

Vanderbilt School of Nursing (2010). *Florence Nightingale pledge*. https://nursing.vanderbilt.edu/news/florence-nightingale-pledge/.

Whittle, D. (1883). I know whom I have believed. In Hymns for the Family of God (1976). Word Music.
Wikipedia Contributors. (2023, November 5). *Peoria State Hospital*. Wikipedia, The Free Encyclopedia.
https://en.wikipedia.org/w/index.php?title=Peoria_State_Hospital&oldid=1183556476.

Wikipedia Contributors. (2024, December 7). *1968 Illinois earthquake*. Wikipedia, The Free Encyclopedia.
https://en.m.wikipedia.org/wiki/1968_Illinois_earthquake.

Wikipedia Contributors. (2024, December 22). *Florence Nightingale*. Wikipedia, The Free Encyclopedia.
https://en.wikipedia.org/wiki,Florence_Nightingale.

www.ingramcontent.com/pod-product-compliance
Lightning Source LLC
Chambersburg PA
CBHW060837170426
43192CB00019BA/2805